D1441089

Conscious Sedation/Analgesia

Donna S. Watson

CONSCIOUS SEDATION/ANALGESIA

Donna S. Watson, RN, MSN, CNOR
**IV Conscious Sedation Consultant and Educator
Fox Island, Washington**

with 41 illustrations

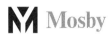

A *Harcourt Health Sciences Company*
St. Louis   Philadelphia   London   Sydney   Toronto

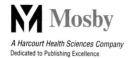

Publisher: Nancy L. Coon
Editor: Michael Ledbetter
Developmental Editor: Nancy L. O'Brien
Project Manager: Deborah L. Vogel
Production Editor: Sarah E. Fike
Design Manager: Pati Pye
Manufacturing Manager: Don Carlisle

A NOTE TO THE READER

The authors and publisher have made every attempt to check dosages and nursing content for accuracy. Because the science of pharmacology is continually advancing, our knowledge base continues to expand. Therefore we recommend that the reader always check product information for changes in dosage or administration before administering any medication. This is particularly important with new or rarely used drugs.

Printed in the United States of America

Mosby–Year Book, Inc.
11830 Westline Industrial Drive
St. Louis, Missouri 63146

Library of Congress Cataloging-in-Publication Data

Watson, Donna, MSN.
    Conscious sedation/analgesia / Donna S. Watson. — 1st ed.
      p.   cm.
    Includes bibliographical references and index.
    ISBN 0-8151-9265-7
    1. Conscious sedation. 2. Analgesia. 3. Nurses.   I. Title.
    [DNLM: 1. Conscious Sedation—nursing. 2. Analgesia—nursing.
WY 150 W3369c 1997]
RD85.C64W38   1997
617.9′6—dc21
DNLM/DLC
                                 97-34261

00 01 / 9 8 7 6 5 4

Contributors

Linda Brazen, RN, CNS, MS(N), CNOR,C
Clinical Director and
   Clinical Nurse Specialist
Children's Hospital
Denver, Colorado
(Chapter VII)

Katherine Kay Brown, RN, MSN, CCRN
Cardiothoracic and Vascular Clinical
   Nurse Specialist
Allegheny General Hospital
Assistant Professor of Nursing
Duquesne University
Pittsburgh, Pennsylvania
(Chapter IV)

Tim Sheard, RN, BSN, MA
Teaching and Research Nurse
SUNY Hospital/Downstate
Brooklyn, New York
Faculty, Cross Country University
Faculty, Colleague Medical
(Chapter IX)

Consultants

Ann Fagerness, RN
Director
Health Education Network
Seattle, Washington

Mary Madsen, RN, BSN
Staff Nurse
Methodist Hospital
Brooklyn, New York

Laureen Talenti
Critical Care Consultant/Educator
Enfield, Connecticut

Reviewers

Marianne S. Baird, RN, MN,
CCRN
Case Manager/Clinical Nurse
Specialist
St. Joseph's Hospital of Atlanta
Atlanta, Georgia

Ellen Carson, RNCS, PhD
Associate Professor, Department
of Nursing
Pittsburg State University
Pittsburg, Kansas

Donna M. DeFazio-Quinn, RN,
BSN, MBA, CPAN, CAPA
Elliot One-Day Surgery Center
(a subsidiary of Optima Health)
Manchester, New Hampshire

Sandra L. Dunn, RN, CNOR,
BSEd
O.R. Clinical Educator
St. Luke's Hospital Medical Center
(an OrNda facility)
Phoenix, Arizona

Cheri Goll, RN, MSN
Assistant Program Director
Indiana University Medical Center
Indianapolis, Indiana

Donna Jensen, RN, MPH, CCRN
Staff Nurse, Adult Critical Care
University of Minnesota Hospital
and Clinic
Minneapolis, Minnesota

Antoinette K. Ledbetter, RN, MS,
CNOR
Trauma Services
St. John's Mercy Medical Center
St. Louis, Missouri

Suzan W. New, RN, BSN, CNOR
Leadership Development
Consultant
Baylor Health Care System
Dallas, Texas

K. Sue Phillips, RN, BS, MS,
CNOR
Perioperative Coordinator
Carle Foundation Hospital
Urbana, Illinois

Preface

This book provides a guide for a safe standard of care for the patient receiving conscious sedation/analgesia. The information included is based on national recommended practices, guidelines, and position statements from various nursing and medical organizations. This book is intended for the registered nurse (RN) who is responsible for managing the care of a patient receiving conscious sedation/analgesia during a short-term therapeutic, diagnostic, or surgical procedure.

Chapter I provides essential information for the RN. It highlights the *Association of Operating Room Nurses Recommended Practices for Managing the Patient Receiving Conscious Sedation/ Analgesia;* the *Position Statement on the Role of the Registered Nurse (RN) in the Management of Patients Receiving IV Conscious Sedation for Short-Term Therapeutic, Diagnostic, or Surgical Procedures;* the *American Society of Anesthesiologists Practice Guidelines for Sedation and Analgesia by Non-Anesthesiologists;* the *American Association of Nurse Anesthetists Position Statement: Qualified Providers of Conscious Sedation,* and various statements from state boards of nursing regarding the role and responsibilities of RNs in their respective states. This chapter is critical in establishing an institutional standard of care that defines expected nursing responsibilities and the quality of care that a patient receiving conscious sedation and analgesia should receive.

Chapter II focuses on what is expected of the RN in regard to patient monitoring. Chapter III presents a quick reference of medications commonly administered for conscious sedation/analgesia. Chapter IV is dedicated to the management of complications potentially associated with conscious sedation/analgesia. Other topics included in this book are patient discharge (Chapter V), development of institutional guidelines (Chapter VI), and competency issues (Chapter VII). The chapters on pediatric sedation (Chapter VIII) and the critically ill patient (Chapter IX) present the latest techniques and recommended guidelines for the proper management of these special populations.

Recently there has been an increase in published material concerning the role of the RN in managing the care of the patient receiving conscious sedation/analgesia. The goal of this book is to provide a summary of the expected roles and responsibilities for the RN based on national guidelines and state boards of nursing statements. Because variations in practice do occur in the delivery of care to the patient receiving conscious sedation/analgesia, I have made the focus of this book positive patient outcomes. Through implementation of appropriate monitoring parameters and adherence to the guidelines recommended throughout this book, the RN can significantly lower the risk of an untoward patient outcome and achieve a high quality of patient care.

Donna S. Watson

This book is dedicated to my family—Bob, Chris, and Danny

Acknowledgments

I would like to thank my nursing colleagues, who have provided me with the support and encouragement to write a book on conscious sedation/analgesia. As with any project, it is never accomplished alone, and I could not have completed the book without the assistance of the contributors. I thank all of you for the wonderful work and significant contributions you have made. Thank you to Katherine Kay Brown for addressing the complications associated with conscious sedation/analgesia (Chapter IV); to Linda Brazen for writing about competence in managing the patient receiving conscious sedation/analgesia (Chapter VII); and to Tim Sheard for discussing sedation in the mechanically ventilated patient (Chapter IX).

I also want to thank Michael Ledbetter and Nancy O'Brien from Mosby and Carlotta Seely from Top Graphics for believing in this project and for the encouragement and often needed support.

Last, I would like to thank my husband, Bob, who spent many days, evenings, and nights with the boys so that I was able to give this book my full attention. Also, Chris and Danny, I thank you for being my guiding light.

Donna S. Watson

Contents

Appendixes

History of Conscious Sedation

In recent years outpatient surgery has drastically increased because of advances in technology, pharmacology, and anesthesia technique. In 1995 close to 4 million procedures were performed at outpatient surgery centers in the United States. By the year 2000 approximately 70% of patient care will be provided in alternative settings, such as physicians' offices or free-standing facilities (Michel & Myrick, 1990). Today the anesthetic technique of choice for a significant portion of outpatient surgery is intravenous conscious sedation and analgesia. Many physicians, nurses, and patients prefer the administration of conscious sedation and analgesia over general anesthesia for patients who meet appropriate selection criteria. In the future an increase in the administration of conscious sedation and analgesia over general anesthesia can be expected for specific short-term therapeutic, diagnostic, and surgical procedures.

One of the main advantages of conscious sedation and analgesia is the patient's rapid return to presedation levels: such patients generally experience a shorter recovery period, ambulate earlier, and more readily participate in the discharge process than do patients receiving general anesthesia. Side effects from the medications are minimal and complications are few.

At issue is determining the most appropriate provider to administer and monitor the patient receiving conscious sedation and analgesia. The demand for such anesthesia providers is greater than the supply, resulting in an increased use of nonanesthesia providers to administer conscious sedation and analgesia. The nonanesthesia provider is generally a professional registered nurse (RN) who receives additional training in administering conscious sedation and analgesia medications and monitoring the patient. In some instances the nonanesthesia provider is a technician and not an RN. Issues concerning the role and use of the nonanesthesia provider include appropriateness of allowing health care providers who are not specifically trained and educated in the techniques of anesthesia to administer conscious sedation and analgesia medications; determining the competency of the health care provider; selecting patients based on identified criteria; identifying types of medications that may be administered safely by the nonanesthesia provider; and identifying appropriate levels of sedation and types of procedures with few predicted complications (Box 1-1).

BOX 1-1 *Procedures Performed With Patient Under Conscious Sedation and Analgesia and Monitored by Nonanesthesia RNs**

Head and neck procedures
  Molar extractions
  Blepharoplasty
  Rhytidoplasty
  Rhinoplasty
  Laceration repair
  Cataract extraction
Superficial thoracic procedures
  Breast augmentation
  Breast biopsy
  Bronchoscopy
  Chest tube insertion
Extremity procedures
  Carpal tunnel release
  Trigger finger release
  Removal of pins/wires/screws
  Closed reduction
Gastrointestinal abdominal procedures
  Endoscopic retrograde
    cholangiopancreatography

Colonoscopy
Endoscopic ultrasonography
Gastroscopy
Vascular procedures
  Hemodialysis access placement
  Pacemaker insertion
  Angiography
  Cardiac catheterization
  Radiofrequency ablation
  Electrophysiologic testing
Gynecologic/urologic procedures
  Dilatation and curettage
  Fulguration vaginal lesions
  Fulgration anal lesions
  Cystoscopy
  Incision and drainage of Bartholin's cyst
  Vasectomy

*This list of examples is not intended to be all-inclusive.

HISTORY—NURSING PERSPECTIVE

Conscious sedation is a technique that originated in the practices of oral surgery and dentistry (Kallar, 1991; Nemiroff, 1993). It is popular and widely used to supplement local or regional anesthesia during a variety of short-term, therapeutic, and diagnostic procedures. Many patients prefer the light sleep of conscious sedation and analgesia versus general anesthesia and like the added amnesic benefit that many of the medications provide. The goals of patient care are to provide adequate analgesia and sedation safely, while allaying patient fears and anxiety.

During the 1980s the RN's primary technique of conscious sedation and analgesia included administering a benzodiazepine (i.e., diazepam) and/or narcotic (i.e., meperidine) for the adequate control and management of pain versus sedation (Mauldin, 1986). Procedures were relatively low risk, and patients were usually young and healthy with no other preexisting illness. The parameters monitored during the procedure varied and generally included blood pressure, heart rate, and respiration. Patient assessment findings and monitoring parameters were documented at 15- to 30-

minute intervals. One RN was assigned to the patient and had circulating and monitoring responsibilities. The patient was transported for recovery to the postanesthesia care unit (PACU) and monitored in the same way as a patient receiving general anesthesia. The patient was then discharged home or transferred to a nursing unit.

Today's very different scenario can be attributed to the continual increase in ambulatory surgery, reimbursement regulations, and consumer demand. Patients are demanding painless surgery with the latest technology, and they expect only minimal disruption in their daily lives during the recovery phase. Many surgical inpatient procedures that formerly required several days of hospitalization have been replaced by minimally invasive outpatient procedures performed in units outside the traditional operating room.

Third-party payers, private insurers, and Medicare closely monitor billing submitted for monitored anesthesia care (MAC). Each carrier determines the types of procedures and patient criteria allowable for reimbursement of services rendered by anesthesia personnel. The result is a change in business as usual.

Significant change is occurring in the provision of MAC. The American Society of Anesthesiologists (1994) defines MAC as:

> Instances in which an anesthesiologist has been called upon to provide specific anesthesia services to a particular patient undergoing a planned procedure, in connection with which a patient receives local anesthesia, or in some cases, no anesthesia at all. In such a case, the anesthesiologist is providing specific services to the patient and is in control of his or her nonsurgical or nonobstetrical medical care, including the responsibility of monitoring his or her vital signs, and is available to administer anesthetics or provide other medical care as appropriate (p. 37).

In the past anesthesia providers were responsible for MAC. Presently at many institutions MAC is the responsibility of an RN or a technician. It has been suggested that in some instances this additional responsibility may border on the practice of anesthesia without proper education.

This situation raises many questions and issues regarding the nonanesthesia provider's responsibility for monitoring and/or administering medications for conscious sedation and analgesia. The newer medications are close to ideal: they are of short duration, are rapid acting, can be administered through a variety of routes, and have greater predictability and fewer side effects. However, the one significant disadvantage of the newer medications is the increasing difficulty of determining if the patient is approaching the outer boundaries of conscious sedation and analgesia (i.e., unconsciousness). The patient may be responsive and talking while the monitoring parameters indicate that the patient is experiencing mild hypoxemia. Some nonanesthesia providers administer anesthetic medications that are manufactured for use in general anesthesia. This improper administration of these medications can rapidly induce the patient to a level of deep sedation or general anesthesia, a state clearly beyond the scope of practice for the nonanesthesia provider.

One area that has been difficult to define is the acceptable standard of care to be provided by the nonanesthesia provider. The growing expectation is that the nonanesthesia provider should be held to the same standard of care as are anesthesia personnel—that is, the American Society of Anesthesiology "Standards for Basic Anesthetic Monitoring" (see Appendix B). Aker and Rupp (1994) state, "Standards do *not* vary according to the type of practitioner that provides it [care]" (p. 94). The patient should not receive a lesser standard of care when conscious sedation and analgesia is administered and/or monitored by a nonanesthesia provider under the direction of a physician with little training and experience in the practice of anesthesia. As nonanesthesia providers participate in the monitoring and/or administering of medications that produce a state of sedation and analgesia, it is imperative that they demonstrate competence and that they provide services within an accepted scope of practice—one that does not extend to the practice of anesthesia.

SCOPE OF PRACTICE ISSUES

As RNs continue to define and refine their role as providers of conscious sedation and analgesia, they have consulted with their state boards of nursing regarding patient care. Consequently several state nursing boards have developed advisory opinions, position statements, declaratory rulings, or guidelines (see Appendix A) to ensure that the RN is capable, experienced, and competent to provide safe patient care. The responses issued by state boards of nursing assist in preventing inappropriate use of nursing staff who are not trained in anesthesia practice or with little experience in the administration of agents of conscious sedation and analgesia. The movement toward the involvement of each state will focus concern on the safety and welfare of the patient.

State Boards of Nursing

Many RNs managing the care of a patient receiving conscious sedation and analgesia rely on administrative authorities to develop a standard of care (i.e., policy and procedures) to guide their daily practice. Often the result is the development of policies and procedures that meet the needs of nursing's colleagues but not necessarily those of the RN or the patient. This situation has prompted many RNs to request assistance from individual state boards of nursing to define acceptable practices for the nonanesthesia RN administering conscious sedation and analgesia. Every RN managing the care of patients receiving conscious sedation and analgesia should keep current on information about this subject issued by his/her state board of nursing.

Table 1-1 presents survey information from each state about the status of the nonanesthesia RN administering conscious sedation (Watson, 1995). The survey results are summarized as follows:

- Overall consensus on the definition of conscious sedation to include the fact that the patient must "independently maintain a patent airway, and be able to respond appropriately to physical stimulation and/or verbal command."

- Five states issued declaratory rulings (i.e., Iowa, Maryland, Montana, New Hampshire, and South Dakota).
- All states responding to the survey found that the administration and monitoring of conscious sedation and analgesia was within the scope of practice for the nonanesthesia RN.
- Seven states refer to the ability of the RN to demonstrate competency of specific skills and knowledge needed to administer conscious sedation and analgesia (i.e., Arkansas, Idaho, Maryland, Nebraska, New York, North Dakota, and Texas).
- Wisconsin and Colorado consider the administration of conscious sedation and analgesia a delegated medical act that may be performed by the RN if the requirements in the rules for the performance of the delegated medical act are met.
- Arkansas, California, Colorado, Idaho, Kansas, Maryland, Nebraska, New York, North Dakota, Vermont, and West Virginia support the position statement endorsed by 23 specialty nursing organizations (see Appendix C).

The RN managing the care of a patient receiving conscious sedation and analgesia should periodically consult the state board of nursing for any recent and relevant information. Institution policies and procedures should be consistent with the state board of nursing's recommendations, which reflect current practice. Table 1-1 shows a summary of the study results.

Standards of Practice

Several resources can be used to develop the standards of practice for the RN who manages the care of a patient receiving conscious sedation and analgesia. These resources include state board of nursing statutes; professional organization position statements, guidelines, and recommended practices; literature review; and actual practices occurring in an institution. Often the practices followed in an institution fall below the national standards set by professional organizations. It is important for institutions and the RN managing the care of a patient receiving conscious sedation and analgesia to be knowledgeable about national standards and recommendations, which are used in courts of law to determine malpractice or negligence.

The American Nurses Association (ANA) recognized the need for nursing standards in the 1960s. In 1965 the ANA Committee on Nursing Services developed the first nursing standards for organized nursing services (Flanagan, 1976). In 1973 the ANA published the first standards for nursing practice. These generic nursing standards were specific to the practice of nursing, based on the nursing process, and intended to apply to every RN. Since that time many specialty nursing organizations have promulgated their own nursing standards, resulting in confusion caused by the lack of consistency in definitions, intent, and format.

In 1991, nearly two decades after issuing its first standards, the ANA published revised standards for nursing practice. These generic standards are intended to apply to every practicing RN. The ANA collaborated with specialty nursing organizations

TABLE 1-1 *Summary of 1995 Survey on Conscious Sedation*

STATE	COMMENTS	CONSCIOUS SEDATION STATEMENT
Arkansas	Supports position statement (see Appendix C).	Position statement
California	Supports position statement (see Appendix C).	Policy
Colorado	Supports position statement (see Appendix C).	None
Idaho	Non-CRNAs may not administer ketamine. Supports position statement (see Appendix C).	Statement
Iowa	No comments provided.	Declaratory ruling
Kansas	Supports position statement (see Appendix C).	Position statement
Kentucky	In progress of evaluating. Non-CRNAs are not allowed to administer anesthetic agents: ketamine, sodium pentothal, methohexital, and nitrous oxide.	None
Louisiana	Nurse practice act prohibits RNs who are non-CRNAs from administering anesthetic agents.	Statement
Maryland	Non-CRNAs are prohibited from administering ketamine, sodium pentothal, methohexital, propofol, etomidate, and nitrous oxide. Supports position statement (see Appendix C).	Declaratory ruling
Mississippi	No comments provided.	Statement
Missouri	No comments provided.	Opinion on nurse-client situation
Montana	No comments provided.	Declaratory ruling
Nebraska	Supports position statement (see Appendix C).	Position statement
Nevada	Included Nevada State Board of Nursing Practice opinion process.	None
New Hampshire	No comments provided.	Declaratory ruling on administration of midazolam (Versed)
New York	Supports position statement (see Appendix C).	None
North Carolina	No comments provided.	Statement
North Dakota	Supports position statement (see Appendix C).	Opinion
Ohio	Until July 1994 the board of nursing had statements related to intravenous conscious sedation and analgesia. However, the board no longer issues statements and is in the process of developing rule language for standards of nursing care.	None

Modified from Watson, D. Conscious sedation survey. Unpublished research.
CRNAs, Noncertified registered nurse anesthetists; ANA, American Nurses Association; AANA, American Association of Nurse Anesthetists.

TABLE 1-1 *Summary of 1995 Survey on Conscious Sedation—cont'd*

STATE	COMMENTS	CONSCIOUS SEDATION STATEMENT
Oregon	A task force is being convened to discuss the issue.	None
Pennsylvania	No comments provided.	Statement of policy
South Dakota	Adopted position statement (see Appendix C).	Declaratory ruling
Texas	Non-CRNAs are allowed to administer anesthetics and analgesics only for conscious sedation and analgesia, not for complete anesthesia.	Position statement
Vermont	The state board of nursing follows the recommendations of the position statement endorsed by the ANA (see Appendix C).	None
Virginia	CRNAs are separately licensed and their practice is defined and protected; it would be inappropriate for a non-CRNA to administer agents for the sole purpose of anesthesia.	None
West Virginia	The state board of nursing refers to the position statement endorsed by the ANA (see Appendix C) and the AANA position statement (see Appendix D).	None
Wisconsin	Conscious sedation and analgesia is considered a delegated medical act that may be performed by the RN.	Administrative code
Florida, Georgia, Indiana, Maine, Michigan, Minnesota, Oklahoma, Utah; Alabama, Alaska, Arizona, Connecticut, Delaware, District of Columbia, Hawaii, Illinois, Massachusetts, New Jersey, New Mexico, Rhode Island, South Carolina, Tennessee, Washington	No comments provided.	None

in making these revisions and in devising a framework for these organizations to use to develop criteria for specialty nursing standards (e.g., operating room, emergency department, postanesthesia care unit). This collaboration between specialty nursing organizations and the ANA ensures more consistent interpretation of nursing standards. In addition, work was begun on the process of developing future national nursing guidelines (Marek, 1995).

The RN managing the care of the patient receiving conscious sedation and analgesia should clearly understand nursing standards and how they are used to define the RN's scope of practice. A standard describes an expected level of nursing care; there is little room for variation in practice. Under similar circumstances all RNs are expected to exercise the same sound judgment reflected in the standards of care. For example, every RN is expected to provide a plan of care for the patient based on assessment, diagnosis, outcome identification, planning, implementation, and evaluation. Simply stated, standards are "authoritative statements that describe the responsibilities for which nursing practitioners are accountable" (AORN, 1996, p. 97). The ANA's *Standards of Clinical Nursing Practice* includes "Standards of Care" and "Standards of Professional Performance" (Box 1-2), which outline expected knowledge, skills, and professional behavior for the RN.

Professional nursing organizations are responsible for the development and dissemination of acceptable standards of practice. The RN administering conscious sedation and analgesia during short-term therapeutic, diagnostic, or surgical procedures should be conversant with pertinent research published in professional nursing and medical journals. These publications reflect current trends in practice that institutions use to develop policy and procedures for the RN's care of patients receiving conscious sedation and analgesia. The memberships of several associations consist of RNs who manage the care of patients receiving conscious sedation and

---

BOX 1-2 *American Nurses Association Standards of Clinical Nursing Practice*

STANDARDS OF CARE	STANDARDS OF PROFESSIONAL PERFORMANCE
Assessment	Quality of care
Diagnosis	Performance appraisal
Outcome identification	Education
Planning	Collegiality
Implementation	Ethics
Evaluation	Collaboration
	Research
	Resource utilization

Data from American Nurses Association (1991). *Standards of clinical nursing practice* (p.2). Washington, DC: Author.

analgesia on a routine basis (e.g., Association of Operating Room Nurses, American Association of Nurse Anesthetists, Society for Gastrointestinal Nurses and Associates, American Society of PeriAnesthesia Nurses, and American Association of Critical Care Nurses). Each of these nursing associations has published relevant recommended practices, position statements, guidelines, and articles that reflect the latest trends and techniques for safe administration of conscious sedation and analgesia.

In addition, many other nursing and medical associations have been active in the development or endorsement of practice guidelines, position statements, or recommended practices for managing the care of a patient receiving conscious sedation and analgesia (Box 1-3). Each professional association contributes to the development of acceptable practice standards. However, widespread confusion persists concerning who is responsible for monitoring the patient, identification of minimal monitoring parameters, and which standards should be absolute (Fleischer, 1989, 1990; Holzman et al., 1994; Nelson, 1993). Much of this confusion is due to the inconsistent interpretation of position statements, practice guidelines, and recommended practices. A clearer understanding of the intent and purpose is needed before a national standard of care can be developed for the patient receiving conscious sedation and analgesia.

BOX 1-3 *Professional Associations With Endorsements or Positions on Conscious Sedation and Analgesia Administration*

American Academy of Pediatrics
American Association of Neuroscience Nurses
American Association of Nurse Anesthetists
American Association of Spinal Cord Injury Nurses
American Association of Occupational Health Nurses
American Association of Oral and Maxillofacial Surgeons
American Dental Society of Anesthesiology
American Nephrology Nurses Association
American Nurses Association
American Radiological Nurses Association
American Society of Anesthesiologists
American Society of Pain Management Nurses
American Society of Plastic and Reconstructive Surgical Nurses

American Urological Association, Allied
Association of Pediatric Oncology Nurses
Association of Rehabilitation Nurses
Dermatology Nurses Association
Nurses Association of the American College of Obstetricians and Gynecologists
National Association of Orthopaedic Nurses
National Flight Nurses Association
National Student Nurses Association
North American Society of Pacing and Electrophysiology
Nurse Consultants Association, Inc.
Nurses Organization of Veterans Affairs
Nursing Pain Association

Position Statements

Position statements are issued by specialty nursing organizations, state boards of nursing, or other professional associations on actual or emerging practice trends (e.g., conscious sedation and analgesia, patient and health care workers with human immunodeficiency virus, unlicensed assistive personnel). Position statements are developed by a panel of experts. Generally a position statement is based on a professional consensus of the developing group. Because practice is an emerging trend, little scientific research is usually available. Instead, recommendations are based on current practice trends and safe implementation. The position statement may be brief or may outline suggested implementation criteria. Position statements are generally developed because of concern for an area of practice that may be detrimental to patient safety.

The "Position Statement on the Role of the Registered Nurse (RN) in the Management of Patients Receiving IV Conscious Sedation for Short-Term Therapeutic, Diagnostic, or Surgical Procedures" is significant to all RNs managing the care of patients receiving conscious sedation and analgesia (see Appendix C). This position statement has had tremendous impact on the implementation and delivery of nursing care provided to the patient receiving conscious sedation and analgesia. It is frequently referenced by state boards of nursing, state nursing associations, and specialty nursing associations.

The statement resulted from practice concerns expressed by the American Association of Nurse Anesthetists at the November 1990 meeting of the Nursing Organization Liaison Forum (Pashley, 1991). In January 1991 the first discussion group was convened by the ANA at the National Federation for Specialty Nursing Organizations. The goal was to develop a position statement describing specific recommendations for the safe administration of conscious sedation and analgesia by the RN. The final position statement was made available in the fall of 1991 and included the endorsement of 23 specialty nursing organizations. Today many state boards of nursing endorse the position statement or reference it when nursing practice opinions on conscious sedation and analgesia are requested (see Appendix C).

Practice Guidelines

Practice guidelines are "systematically developed statements to assist practitioner and patient decisions about appropriate health care for specific clinical conditions" (Acute Pain Management Guideline Panel, 1992). Guidelines are developed by organizations such as the Agency for Health Care Policy and Research (AHCPR), health care professional organizations, pharmaceutical companies, and other organizations such as private research organizations. The basic criteria for development of guidelines includes that they be "science-based, documented, unbiased, and clear" (Lohr, 1995, p. 50). Nearly a thousand practice guidelines or practice parameters exist, but relatively few meet the criteria suggested by Lohr.

One example of practice guidelines is the revised "Guidelines for Cardiopulmonary Resuscitation and Emergency Cardiac Care" developed by the Emergency Cardiac Care Committee/Subcommittees and American Heart Association (1992). These practice guidelines are part of the curriculum for the American Heart Association's Advanced Cardiac Life Support (ACLS) course. Guidelines such as these are advisory in nature and are not intended to be the only approach to patient management of the clinical problem. The intent is to guide practice while allowing for deviation when necessary.

Implementation of practice guidelines is optional and may include full or partial implementation, or none at all. Practice guidelines are recommended options; they are considered as emerging standards of practice that may eventually become mandated. Guidelines may be used in a legal suit to determine acceptable practice.

Practice guidelines have been taken seriously at the federal level through the approval of the Omnibus Budget Reconciliation Act of 1989, which provides funding for the development of national guidelines through AHCPR. The AHCPR guideline "Acute Pain Management: Operative or Medical Procedures and Trauma" (1992) applies to the RN administering conscious sedation and analgesia, and it details suggested management of pain. The guidelines are revised to reflect current clinical practice and available scientific data. Suggested approaches to pain assessment are discussed in detail in Chapter 3.

The American Dental Society of Anesthesiology and the American Association of Oral and Maxillofacial Surgeons have published guidelines on the administration of conscious sedation and analgesia that are similar to the American Academy of Pediatrics "Guidelines for Monitoring and Management of Pediatric Patients During and After Sedation for Diagnostic and Therapeutic Procedures" described in Chapter 8. The American Association of Nurse Anesthetists has "Suggested Guidelines for Registered Professional Nurses Engaged in the Administration of IV Conscious Sedation" (see Appendix D), and more recently the American Society of Anesthesiologists (1995) adopted "Guidelines for Sedation and Analgesia by Non-anesthesiologists" (see Appendix E).

These recommended guidelines for the administration of conscious sedation and analgesia are developed by medical and nursing organizations that represent professionals involved in the administration of conscious sedation and analgesia. This gives the guidelines a great deal of credibility. Each guideline includes a recommended set of criteria and should be viewed as clinically flexible. The strength of each guideline is verified by supporting evidence. Many associations maintain extensive lists of pertinent literature for their members. It is up to the individual practitioner and institution to choose the most appropriate implementation from interventions and monitoring parameters suggested by the guideline.

Recommended Practices

Recommended practices such as those available from the Association of Operating Room Nurses (AORN) represent nursing consensus on various clinical conditions and technical components of patient care. Recommended practices are statements "intended to represent optimum achievable performance in a practice setting" (Gregory, 1990). They are based on current nursing practice, available scientific data, and standards and regulations from agencies such as the Joint Commission on Accreditation of Healthcare Organizations (JCAHO) and the Occupational Safety and Health Administration (OSHA). Recommended practices serve as guidelines for nursing practice.

The AORN has been in the forefront of advocating safe practices for the perioperative nurse managing the care of the patient receiving intravenous conscious sedation and analgesia. In 1992 the proposed Recommended Practices for Monitoring the Patient Receiving Intravenous Conscious Sedation appeared in the *AORN Journal* and were recently revised and approved by the AORN board of directors (Appendix F). In making such recommendations AORN seeks the achievement of optimal care and compliance with practices that are not mandated.

Recommended practices such as those issued by the AORN are optional in terms of implementation and may not always hold up in the legal system. This is based on a case reported by Horty (1995) in which a surgical clamp was left in the abdomen and both the jury and the court of appeals failed to award the patient monetary compensation. However, this case presented some unique occurrences, and one should not infer that recommended practices, position statements, or guidelines do not carry significant weight under the present legal system because they do.

Typically, during a malpractice proceeding related to conscious sedation and analgesia, the previously mentioned guidelines, position statements, recommended practices from national organizations, and recommendations from pharmaceutical companies would be presented as an expected and acceptable standard of care. If the standard of care in the case did not meet the recommendations, the defendant (i.e., RN, technician, physician, or other) would justify and explain exactly how the standard of care delivered was determined. This would include the defendant attempting to justify why national guidelines, position statements, and recommended practices were not implemented and why the care failed to yield to the best interest of the patient.

Development of a Standard of Care

Guidelines, position statements, and recommended practices all contribute to the development of a standard of care (i.e., what the RN is expected to do for the patient). The following suggestions may be helpful in defining a standard of care for the RN who is not trained and educated as an anesthesia provider but is responsible for managing the care of a patient receiving conscious sedation and analgesia:

1. *Contact state board of nursing.* Determine if the administration of conscious sedation and analgesia is within the legal scope of nursing practice for a nonanes-

thesia RN. Are there specific medications that should not be administered by the nonanesthesia RN for purposes of conscious sedation and analgesia in that specific state? Are there any special conditions or criteria that must be in place (e.g., monitoring parameters, required equipment that must be present, continuing education requirements)?

2. *Obtain position statements, guidelines, and recommended practices on the role of the nonanesthesia provider for managing the care of a patient receiving conscious sedation and analgesia from professional associations.* Determine commonalities and differences among the professional associations on issues related to standards of care (e.g., monitoring parameters). Assess and determine which recommendations the institution is willing to implement. Be able to provide a rationale based on continuous quality improvement documentation and scientific data from the literature.

3. *Determine if insurance carriers have specific criteria that must be in place.* Insurance carriers generally do not issue guidelines related to patient care. However, some have issued guidelines for institutions providing conscious sedation and analgesia to patients (St. Paul Fire and Marine Insurance Company Risk Management Services, 1988). Determine if the carrier has such guidelines and implement accordingly.

4. *Assess the standard of care provided to the patient receiving conscious sedation and analgesia.* Does this standard meet the recommendations presented in the national position statements, guidelines, and recommended practices? If not, determine why and evaluate overall patient safety and potential for harm.

5. *Evaluate the different departments administering conscious sedation and analgesia.* Determine if there is a consistent standard of care provided to all patients under similar conditions. If the answer is no, evaluate why the differences exist and correct them according to information found.

LEVELS OF SEDATION

The nonanesthesia provider managing the care of the patient receiving conscious sedation and analgesia should be able to define the different levels of sedation. Sedation occurs on a continuum—with conscious sedation and analgesia at one end and general anesthesia at the other (Figure 1-1). The nonanesthesia provider should be knowledgeable about the differences in the sedation levels and able to determine when the patient is approaching deep sedation or general anesthesia.

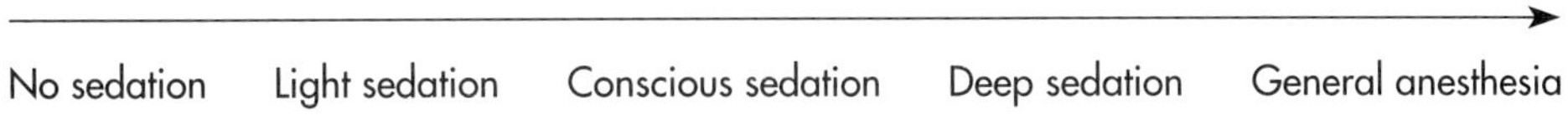

No sedation   Light sedation   Conscious sedation   Deep sedation   General anesthesia

FIGURE 1-1 | Sedation continuum.

The continuum of sedation allows for the patient to progress from one degree to another, based on the medications administered, route, and dosages. "Light sedation" is the administration of oral medications for the reduction of anxiety (e.g., premedication). The patient is technically awake but under the influence of the medication administered. The following statements are applicable to a patient under "light sedation":

1. Protective reflexes are intact (e.g., normal respirations, eye movement, and ability to communicate).
2. The patient does not experience amnesia.
3. The patient's anxiety level and fear are lowered.

A widely accepted definition of conscious sedation and analgesia from the literature is that the patient exhibits a minimally depressed level of consciousness that retains the ability to maintain a patent airway independently and continuously and to respond appropriately to verbal commands and/or physical stimulation (ANA, 1991; AORN, 1996). The clinical characteristics of a patient under conscious sedation and analgesia include the following:

1. Maintenance of protective reflexes (e.g., ability to control secretions, avoiding aspiration, and breathe without assistance)
2. Independent and continuous maintenance of a patent airway
3. Appropriate response to physical stimulation and/or verbal command
4. Easy arousal
5. Minimally depressed level of consciousness
6. Slightly slurred speech

The American Academy of Pediatrics (1992) defines heavy or deep sedation as:

> a medically controlled state of depressed consciousness or unconsciousness from which the patient is not easily aroused. It may be accompanied by a partial or complete loss of protective reflexes, and includes the inability to maintain a patent airway independently and respond purposefully to physical stimulation or verbal command (p. 1110).

The following clinical conditions are indicative of a deeply sedated patient:

1. Not easily aroused
2. Partial or complete loss of protective reflexes
3. Loss of ability to maintain a patent airway independently
4. Unlikely to respond to physical stimulation or verbal command
5. Severely slurred speech

Deep sedation is similar to general anesthesia in that the protective reflexes are lost and the patient is unable to maintain a patent airway and does not respond to physical or verbal comment. Monitoring parameters for deep sedation should be the same as for general anesthesia. The potential for complications increases with deep sedation, and the nonanesthesia provider should avoid managing the care of a patient with one or more clinical indications of deep sedation (Table 1-2). Exceptions to this would occur in areas such as the critical care unit, where the patient is mechanically ventilated and compromised respiratory status rendered by deep sedation is not an issue.

OBJECTIVES OF CONSCIOUS SEDATION

Under the direction of a physician, the RN may be responsible for titrating medications to the patient's response and monitoring the patient under conscious sedation and analgesia. For proper titration the RN should be knowledgeable about the objectives of conscious sedation and analgesia (Bennett, 1984):

1. *The patient's mood should be altered.* Many patients fear general anesthesia and will avoid being "put to sleep" if at all possible. These patients have a high level of fear and apprehension. Many medications alter the patient's mood, allowing for greater acceptance of the procedure about to be performed.

2. *The patient must remain cooperative.* If a patient is uncooperative, it may be impossible to complete the procedure. An anesthesia provider may be requested to place the patient under deep sedation or general anesthesia. If administering conscious sedation and analgesia in conjunction with regional anesthesia, the RN should allow sufficient time for the local anesthetic to take effect after injection (i.e., blockage of nerve impulse).

| TABLE 1-2 | *Differences Between Conscious Sedation and Deep Sedation* |

CONSCIOUS SEDATION	DEEP (UNCONSCIOUS) SEDATION
Mood altered	Patient unconscious
Patient cooperative	Patient unable to cooperate
Protective reflexes intact	Protective reflexes obtunded
Vital signs stable	Vital signs labile
Local anesthesia provides analgesia	Pain eliminated centrally
Amnesia may be present	Amnesia always present
Short recovery room stay	Occasional prolonged recovery; room stay or overnight admission required
Perioperative complications infrequent	Perioperative complications reported in 25%-75% of cases
Uncooperative or mentally disabled patient cannot always be managed	Useful in managing difficult or mentally disabled patients

From Wechtler, B.V. (1988). *Problems in anesthesia.* Philadelphia: J. B. Lippincott.

3. *The pain threshold should be elevated.* As mentioned previously, regional anesthesia may be administered to manage operative pain. However, opioids may also be administered to elevate the pain threshold. Proper patient education is essential. Because it is unlikely that the diagnostic or operative procedure will be pain free, the patient should be aware that tugging, pulling, and discomfort may ensue. The medications simply elevate the pain threshold. Because the technique of conscious sedation and analgesia does not render the patient unconscious, total absence of pain is unlikely.

4. *All protective reflexes should remain active.* A patient with intact protective reflexes should be able to respond to physical and verbal commands. The patient should also be capable of communicating any discomfort or other relevant information to the monitoring RN. Eye movements should be normal. Pharyngeal and laryngeal reflexes (e.g., swallowing, retching, vomiting) should be intact. Respirations should be regular and normal, and the patient should be able to maintain a patent airway without assistance.

5. *There should be only minor deviations in the patient's vital signs.* Only little variation in physiologic monitoring parameters from baseline should be noted. Depending on the method of administration and injection technique (i.e., bolus versus slow titration), there may be some variation in vital signs; however, these are usually only transient and vital signs should return rapidly to baseline.

6. *There may be a degree of amnesia.* The amnesic effect varies with the type of medication and the dosage administered. Certain procedures and diagnostic studies may be recalled as unpleasant experiences for the postanesthesia patient. From this standpoint the amnesic effects rendered by agents such as the benzodiazepines are desirable, especially for the patient who can expect repeated exposures to certain short-term therapeutic, diagnostic, or surgical procedures (e.g., colonoscopy, cardioversion). The nurse responsible for managing the care of the patient should be knowledgeable about every objective and apply them in daily practice. The RN is responsible for monitoring and assessing the patient throughout the procedure or diagnostic study. Continuous patient assessment is important to determine if the objectives of conscious sedation and analgesia are being met (i.e., relaxed and cooperative, slightly slurred speech, easily aroused, patent airway).

PATIENT SELECTION

The ideal patient for conscious sedation and analgesia is one who has received proper education about the procedure and is cooperative. Not all patients are amenable to the techniques of conscious sedation and analgesia; some patients may be more appropriately managed by an anesthesia provider. Patients who have a high level of anxiety, a previous or current history of drug abuse or alcoholism, or post-traumatic stress syndrome and pediatric patients may pose difficulties to the nonanesthesia provider who is administering conscious sedation and analgesia.

Patients should be selected on an individual basis, with consideration given to the existing medical diagnosis, past medical history, age, type of procedure and current history, physical examination, and medical condition. Any of these considerations may increase the risk for an undesirable outcome for the patient under conscious sedation and analgesia. The objective is avoid any patient with an existing complication that may increase the likelihood of a poor outcome. The RN who for any reason does not feel comfortable managing the care of a patient should consult with an anesthesia provider and the attending physician. A joint decision should be made concerning who is the most appropriate person to monitor the patient and the appropriate medications and monitoring parameters to use.

Conscious sedation and analgesia is administered in a variety of settings within an institution. These include, but are not limited to, surgery, PACU, cardiac catheterization laboratory, radiology, emergency department, intensive/coronary care units, cardiac nursing units, electrophysiology department, gastroenterology department, and pain management center. It is not uncommon for a specialty unit to receive a patient who is considered at risk because of a high acuity level (e.g., cardiac insufficiency). If the RN who will be responsible for managing the care of the patient receiving conscious sedation and analgesia does not have the proper training and education to manage the basic care of the patient, it is inappropriate to place the patient under the full management of this RN, even in the immediate presence of a physician. The most appropriate care for such a patient may be provided by an anesthesia provider or an additional RN with the necessary competency to assist in management of the patient's care. The bottom line is safe patient care.

CONCLUSION

The nonanesthesia provider responsible for managing the care of the patient receiving conscious sedation and analgesia should be knowledgeable about national position statements, guidelines, recommended practices, and state board of nursing recommendations. These should be carefully evaluated and integrated into written policies and procedures relating the accepted standard of practice for the given institution. The policies and procedures should be reviewed annually and revised to reflect current practices and scientific principles as available.

REFERENCES

Agency for Health Care Policy and Research, Public Health Services, U.S. Department of Health and Human Services. (February 1992)*, Acute pain management: Operative or medical procedures and trauma. Clinical practice guideline* (AHCPR Pub. No. 92-0032). Rockville, MD: Acute Pain Management Guideline Panel.

Aker, J. G., & Rupp, R. M. (1994). Standards of care in anesthesia practice. In S. D. Foster & L. M. Jorda (Eds.), *Professional aspects of nurse anesthesia practice* (pp. 89-112). Philadelphia: F. A. Davis.

American Academy of Pediatrics Committee on Drugs. (1992). Guidelines for monitoring and management of pediatric patients during and after sedation for diagnostic and therapeutic procedures. *Pediatrics, 22,* 626-627.

American Nurses Association. (1991). *Standards of clinical nursing practice.* Kansas City: Author.

American Society of Anesthesiologists. (1994). *ASA standards, guidelines and statements.* Park Ridge, IL: Author.

American Society of Anesthesiologists. (1995). *Guidelines for sedation and analgesia by non-anesthesiologists.* Park Ridge, IL: Author.

Association of Operating Room Nurses, Inc. (1996). *Standards and recommended practices.* Denver: Author.

Bennett, C. R. (1984). *Monheim's local anesthesia and pain control in dental practice* (7th ed.). St. Louis: Mosby.

Emergency Cardiac Care Committee and Subcommittees, American Heart Association. (1992). Guidelines for cardiopulmonary resuscitation and emergency cardiac care. *JAMA, 268,* 2171-2295.

Flanagan, L. (1976). *One strong voice.* Kansas City: American Nurses Association.

Fleischer, D. (1989). Monitoring the patient receiving conscious sedation. *Gastrointestinal Endoscopy, 35(3),* 262-266.

Fleischer, D. (1990). Monitoring for conscious sedation: perspective of the gastrointestinal endoscopist. *Gastrointestinal Endoscopy, 36* (3 Suppl), S19-22.

Gregory, B. S. (1990). AORN recommended practices: A valuable resource, not policy. *AORN Journal, 52(2),* 361-368.

Holzman, R. S., Cullen, D. J., Eichhorn, J. H., & Philip, J. H. (1994). Guidelines for sedation by nonanesthesiologists during diagnostic and therapeutic procedures. *Journal of Clinical Anesthesia, 6,* 265-276.

Horty, J. (1995). Nurses, surgeon not negligent in retained instrument suit. *OR Manager, 11(3),* 26, 30.

Kallar, S. K., & Dunwiddie, W. C. (1988). Conscious sedation. In BV Wechtler (Ed.), *Problems in anesthesia.* Philadelphia: J. B. Lippincott.

Lohr, K. N. (1995). Guidelines for clinical practice: What they are and why they count. *Journal of Law, Medicine & Ethics, 23,* 49-56.

Marek, K. D. (1995). *Manual to develop guidelines.* Washington, DC: American Nurses Association.

Mauldin, B. (1986). Monitoring patient for local cases: Nursing responsibilities. *AORN Journal, 44(5),* 841-847.

Michel, L. L., & Myrick, C. (1990). Current and future trends in ambulatory surgery and their impact on nursing practice. *Journal of Post Anesthesia Nursing, 5(5),* 347-349.

Nelson, M. D. (1993). Guidelines for monitoring and care of children during and after sedation for imaging studies. *American Journal of Roentgenology, 160,* 581-582.

Nemiroff, M. S. (1993). IV conscious sedation: Essential techniques of monitoring. *Trends in Health Care, Law & Ethics, 8(1),* 87-90.

Pashley, H. (1991). Specialty nursing organizations discuss strategic plans, legislative stance, specialty certification. *AORN Journal, 53(4),* 1062-1064.

St. Paul Fire and Marine Insurance Company Risk Management Services (1988). Medication alert: Versed. *Prism Newsletter, 3,* 1-5.

Watson, D. (1995). Conscious sedation survey. Unpublished research.

Monitoring Parameters and Equipment

Because there is ongoing controversy regarding the monitoring of patients receiving medications for conscious sedation and analgesia, many state boards of nursing are defining specific parameters that must be in place for the registered nurse (RN) managing the care of such patients. Professional organizations such as those described in Chapter 1 periodically update existing position statements, guidelines, and recommended practices that identify specific monitoring parameters. Such parameters are important because they aid the RN in preventing and detecting complications that can have serious consequences for patients.

The RN managing the care of a patient receiving conscious sedation and analgesia is responsible for collecting qualitative and quantitative data. Qualitative data include observations of parameters such as the patient's skin color, depth and character of respirations, movement, pupil size, and sedation level. Quantitative data include physiologic measurements such as blood pressure, respiration rate, heart rate and rhythm, and oxygen saturation. Continuous monitoring of both qualitative and quantitative parameters ensures early detection of complications that may result from the administration of medications or from the procedure. Before the RN administers any medication for conscious sedation and analgesia, the patient should be thoroughly assessed to determine any contraindications or risks that may interfere with a predictable positive patient outcome.

PREPROCEDURE ASSESSMENT

The primary purpose of the preprocedure nursing assessment is to obtain baseline health information and determine preexisting illnesses and conditions that might render nurse-monitored sedation inappropriate. Procedures being performed with the patient under nurse-monitored sedation are becoming increasingly complex with deeper sedative levels and a higher patient acuity level. Every RN responsible for the continuous monitoring of a patient receiving conscious sedation and analgesia should be aware of the instances for which care is more appropriately managed by an anesthesia provider. If the RN determines that it is not in the patient's best interest to be monitored by a nonanesthesia provider, the RN, the physician, and the anesthesia provider should consult to determine the most appropriate person to monitor the patient and the monitoring parameters.

The preprocedure assessment conducted by the RN responsible for monitoring the patient should include data collection from a variety of sources, such as chart review, patient assessment and interview, and consultation with other health care providers as appropriate. The goals of the preprocedure nursing assessment include the following:

1. *Determining appropriate patient selection.* The American Society of Anesthesiologists (ASA) ranks patient physical status on a scale of 1 to 6 (Table 2-1). Although this classification system is used by anesthesia personnel, many institutions also use it to determine patient selection for nurse-monitored sedation. It is common

TABLE 2-1 *Physical (P) Status Classification of the American Society of Anesthesiologists*

STATUS* (SYMBOL)†	DEFINITION	DESCRIPTION AND EXAMPLES
P1	A normal healthy patient	No physiologic, psychologic, biochemical, or organic disturbance
P2	A patient with mild systemic disease	Cardiovascular disease with minimal rest, asthma, chronic bronchitis, obesity, or diabetes mellitus
P3	A patient with severe systemic disease that limits activity but is not incapacitating	Cardiovascular or pulmonary disease that limits activity; severe diabetes with systemic complications; history of myocardial infarction, angina pectoris, or poorly controlled hypertension
P4	A patient with severe systemic disease that is a constant threat to life	Severe cardiac, pulmonary, renal, hepatic, or endocrine dysfunction
P5	A moribund patient who is not expected to survive 24 hours with or without the operation	Surgery is done as last recourse or resuscitative effort; major multisystem or cerebral trauma, ruptured aneurysm, or large pulmonary embolus
P6	A patient declared brain dead whose organs are being removed for donor purposes	

Reprinted with permission of the American Society of Anesthesiologists, 520 N. Northwest Parkway, Park Ridge, IL 60068-2573.

*In status 2, 3, and 4 the systemic disease may or may not be related to the cause for surgery.

†For any patient (P1 through P5) requiring emergency surgery, an *E* is added to the physical status; for example, P1E, P2E. ASA 1 through ASA 6 is often used for physical status.

for patients who are healthy or have a mild systemic disease (e.g., P1 and P2) to be monitored by an RN. In patients with a disease process, the condition must be medically controlled and no contraindications to the sedation/analgesia medications should be present. Patients in the P1 and P2 categories are less likely to develop complications related to the administration of medications for conscious sedation and analgesia or to the procedure itself. Any patient with a systemic disease process (e.g., P3 or higher) should be individually assessed to determine that the systemic disease is medically controlled and stable. There should be no contraindication for the administration of conscious sedation and analgesia medications.

2. *Determining appropriate mental and psychologic status.* The course of the diagnostic, therapeutic, or surgical procedure produces stress and anxiety in most patients. Assessment should include identification of any underlying medical problems (e.g., angina pectoris, sickle cell disease) that may exacerbate during stress. Also, a patient undergoing psychiatric care may take medications that interact with most central nervous system depressants commonly administered for conscious sedation and analgesia. Consultation among the monitoring RN, surgeon, and anesthesia provider may be necessary to determine the most appropriate plan of care.

The RN monitoring the patient throughout the short-term diagnostic, therapeutic, or surgical procedure is responsible for the preprocedure assessment. This assessment should include relevant physical assessment, current medications, allergies and sensitivities, current and past medical history, fasting status, history of substance abuse, history of posttraumatic stress syndrome, present psychologic status, communication ability, and understanding of the procedure and of conscious sedation and analgesia. Physical assessment should include baseline vital signs, height, weight, age, oxygen saturation, and a review of systems. An individualized nursing care plan should be developed by the monitoring RN based on the data collected.

Physical Evaluation

For the patient scheduled to have a surgical procedure, the Joint Commission on Accreditation of Healthcare Organizations (JCAHO) requires a history and physical examination before surgery. This requirement may not be applicable if the procedure is therapeutic or diagnostic. If a medical history and physical are included in the patient's chart, the RN may obtain information as appropriate. Physical evaluation by the monitoring RN should include assessment of the heart, lungs, and airway. This information is necessary to determine any indication of circulation impairment and/or difficulties in breathing. The physician should be notified of any abnormalities, and a 12-lead electrocardiogram should be considered. The skin should be assessed for general appearance and color and to determine if the skin is intact, diaphoretic, cold, warm, jaundiced, pale, or cyanotic. Any bruises or lacerations present should be noted and documented.

The administration of sedation and analgesia medications may interfere with the patient's ability to maintain a patent airway; therefore preprocedure evaluation of the lungs and airway is essential. The lungs should be assessed for any abnormal breath sounds such as rales or wheezing. The airway may be assessed using the Mallampati technique, which is used by anesthesia providers to determine possible intubation difficulty, information of potential value to the monitoring RN. The Mallampati technique categorizes the airway into one of three classes (Dierdorf, 1995):

Class 1: Visualization of the faucial pillars, soft palate, and uvula.

Class 2: Visualization of the faucial pillars and soft palate. The uvula is masked by tongue.

Class 3: Visualization of only the soft palate.

If possible, the patient should be assessed in a sitting position. The patient is directed to open the mouth as wide as possible and protrude the tongue, exposing the faucial pillars and uvula at the tongue base. If the classification exceeds class 1, the physician should be notified regarding the appropriate plan of action (Figure 2-1). This simple precautionary measure alerts the monitoring RN and physician to anticipate difficulty in the event of respiratory depression requiring intubation.

In addition to assessing the heart, lungs and airway, the following questions are pertinent and helpful in the management of the care for the patient receiving conscious sedation and analgesia.

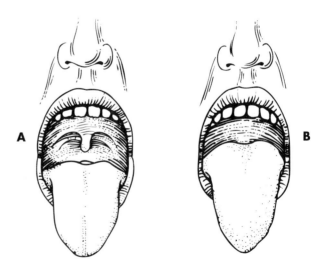

FIGURE 2-1 | Mallampati class 1 airway **(A)** and class 3 airway **(B)**. (From Dierdorf, S. F. [1995]. ASA practice guidelines for management of the difficult airway. *Current Reviews for Nurse Anesthetists,* *17,* 170. Reprinted with permission.)

QUESTION 1

Is there any history of seizure disorder?

Long-term benzodiazepine administration (e.g., diazepam) is often prescribed for patients with convulsive disorders and status epilepticus. Flumazenil, a benzodiazepine antagonist, may be administered to reverse the sedative effects of benzodiazepines. If the patient is undergoing long-term benzodiazepine therapy (e.g., control of intracraneal pressure or status epilepticus) the administration of flumazenil is contraindicated because of the risk of seizures. Research is ongoing in this area, and the practitioner should refer to the scientific literature for further guidance. The potential benefits of the drug should be weighed against the potential risk for these patients.

QUESTION 2

Is there any history of cardiovascular problems?

The RN should evaluate any current or past cardiovascular problem(s) to determine if the patient is at increased risk for developing complications during the procedure while under the effects of conscious sedation and analgesia. Consultation between the monitoring nurse, physician, and anesthesia provider is appropriate to determine the most appropriate provider to monitor the patient.

QUESTION 3

Is there any history of respiratory problems such as emphysema or asthma?

Because many of the medications administered for conscious sedation and analgesia may result in respiratory depression, the patient with an existing respiratory problem is at greater risk for developing complications.

Emphysema is common in patients with bronchitis and asthma. The patient may have a distended barrel-shaped chest and a lower respiratory reserve. A state of chronic hypercarbia exists for patients with chronic obstructive pulmonary disease (e.g., emphysema). The low hypoxic level provides the stimulus for the patient to breathe. Large concentrations of oxygen block the patient's stimulus to breathe. To allow for better control of inspired oxygen fractions and to avoid compromising the drive to breathe in the patient with chronic obstructive pulmonary disease, the RN should consider delivering oxygen via a Venturi mask (Cummins, 1994), which allows for a more precise titration of fixed amounts of oxygen in concentrations of 24%, 28%, 35% and 40%.

The asthmatic patient suffers from attacks of wheezing and dyspnea caused by partial obstruction of the bronchi and bronchioles. The RN should be aware of any causative factors, how the patient manages an episode, and current medications and should have immediately accessible the aerosol inhalant the patient takes to prevent attacks.

Is there any history of liver disease?

RATIONALE

Most of the sedation and analgesia medications administered are metabolized in the liver. The sedative effects may be exaggerated and prolonged because of delayed biotransformation. The extent of liver impairment and the appropriateness of nurse management should be determined by the physician.

QUESTION 5

Is there any history of renal disease?

RATIONALE

Benzodiazepines and narcotic metabolites are excreted in the urine and may be administered with caution to the patient diagnosed with renal insufficiency. The attending physician should be consulted as appropriate.

QUESTION 6

Is there any history of thyroid disorder?

RATIONALE

Hyperthyroidism is not contraindicated for the administration of conscious sedation and analgesia. However, medications such as atropine and local agents administered with epinephrine may further increase the heart rate and precipitate a thyroid crisis. Patients with hyperthyroidism have been found difficult to sedate within normal recommended dosages (Chrisman, et al., 1988; Malamed, 1995). Hypothyroidism may exaggerate the effects of intravenous conscious sedation and analgesia medications. The IV medications should be slowly titrated to the desired effects while the patient is closely monitored. With any thyroid disorder that is medically managed and controlled, the patient should be treated in the same manner as any other patient receiving conscious sedation and analgesia.

QUESTION 7

Is there any history of substance abuse?

RATIONALE

The administration of sedative and analgesia medications may have little or no effect on known substance abusers. Inform the physician and determine a plan of action that includes an anesthesia provider back-up in the event that the patient becomes uncooperative or combative or the medications have little effect on the patient.

QUESTION 8

Are there any known allergies to medications?

RATIONALE

Although a true allergic reaction to a medication is infrequent, the RN should investigate any adverse reaction that a patient describes as an allergy (e.g., rash, pruritus, nausea, vomiting, dizziness, headache). Smith and Petty (1988) identify the following predisposing factors as increasing the patient's risk of developing an adverse reaction: elderly age group, female gender, severe underlying disease, previous medication allergy, hepatic dysfunction, renal failure, inherited enzyme deficiencies, and concomitant drug administration. For each medication administered the RN should be knowledgeable about the effects, contraindications, recommended dosage, potential complications, and populations at increased risk for reactions.

QUESTION 9

Are there any current medications?

RATIONALE

The current medication therapy can be reviewed to determine possible drug-drug interactions when these drugs are administered with sedative agents (Table 2-2).

QUESTION 10

What is the patient's fasting status?

RATIONALE

The ASA recommends (1995) that an adult patient may have solids and nonclear liquids up to 6 to 8 hours before the procedure and clear liquids up to 2 to 3 hours before the procedure (Box 2-1). There should be sufficient time for gastric emptying to occur. When fasting requirements established by an institution are not met by the patient, the potential harm to the patient must be weighed against proceeding with the procedure while the patient is under the effects of conscious sedation and analgesia.

TABLE 2-2	*Drug-Drug Interactions Involving Sedative/Anesthetic Drugs*	
DRUG ACTION	INTERACTING AGENT	RESULTING ACTION
Anesthetics, general	Antidepressants	Hypotension
	Antihypertensives	Hypotension
Barbiturates	Alcohol	Enhanced sedation; ↑respiratory depression
	Anticoagulants, oral	↓Anticoagulant, effect
	Antidepressants	↓Antidepressant effect
	β-Adrenergic blockers	↓β-blocker effect
	Corticosteroids	↓Steroid effect
	Digitalis	↓Digitalis effect
	Doxycycline	↓Doxycycline effect
	Griseofulvin	↓Griseofulvin effect
	Phenothiazines	↓Phenothiazine effect
	Quinidine	↓Quinidine effect
	Rifampin	↓Barbiturate effect
	Valproic acid	↓Phenobarbital effect
Benzodiazepines	Alcohol	Enhanced sedation
	Barbiturates	Enhanced sedation; ↑respiratory depression
Meperidine	Barbiturates	↑Central nervous system depression
	Curariform drugs	↑Respiratory depression
	Monoamine oxidase inhibitors (MAOIs)	Hypertension
Phenothiazines	Alcohol	↑Sedation
	Guanethidine	↓Phenothiazine effect
	Levodopa	↓Levodopa effect
	Lithium	↓Phenothiazine effect
Sympathomimetic amines (epinephrine)	Antidepressants	Hypertension, hypertensive crisis
	Antihypertensives	↓Antihypertensive effect
	β-Adrenergic blockers	Hypertension with epinephrine
	Halogenated anesthetics	Cardiac dysrhythmias with epinephrine
	Digitalis drugs	↑Cardiac dysrhythmias
	Indomethacin	Severe hypertension
	MAOIs	Hypertensive crisis

Modified from ADA Council on Dental Therapeutics. (1983). Clinical products in dentistry, *Journal of the American Dental Association, 107*, 885.

BOX 2-1 *Example of Fasting Protocol for Conscious Sedation and Analgesia With Elective Procedures*

Gastric emptying may be influenced by many factors including anxiety, pain, abnormal autonomic function (e.g., diabetes), pregnancy, and mechanical obstruction. Therefore the suggestions below do not guarantee that complete gastric emptying has occurred. Unless contraindicated, pediatric patients should be offered clear liquids until 2 to 3 hours before sedation to minimize the risk of dehydration.

	SOLIDS AND NONCLEAR LIQUIDS*	CLEAR LIQUIDS
Adults	6-8 hr or none after midnight†	2-3 hr
Children >36 mo	6-8 hr	2-3 hr
Children 6-36 mo	6 hr	2-3 hr
Children <6 mo	4-6 hr	2 hr

*This includes milk, formula, and breast milk (high fat content may delay gastric emptying).
†There are no data to establish whether a 6 to 8 hour fast is equivalent to an overnight fast prior to sedation/analgesia.
From *American Society of Anesthesiologists guidelines for sedation and analgesia by non-anesthesiologists.* Reprinted with permission of the American Society of Anesthesiologists, 520 N. Northwest Parkway, Park Ridge, IL 60068-2573.

INTRAPROCEDURAL MONITORING

Controversy about universal versus selective monitoring is ongoing. Issues that continue to be unresolved include the following: Should a patient undergoing an endoscopic procedure be monitored differently than a patient undergoing a surgical procedure or a patient in the emergency department? Should a history and physical examination be required for every patient who will receive conscious sedative and analgesia medications? What is minimal laboratory work that should be done? What are minimal documentation intervals? Should the RN and the physician be certified in advanced cardiac life support? What is the minimal fasting status for the patient undergoing conscious sedation and analgesia? Should the patient be monitored with an electrocardiogram (ECG)?

Often the decisions that determine which monitoring parameters are implemented is based on projected cost of the equipment and personnel. Until there is scientific data to support the exclusion of a specific monitoring parameter, minimal monitoring parameters for the patient receiving conscious sedation and analgesia should include continuous assessment of pulmonary ventilation, oxygenation, blood pressure, cardiac rate and rhythm, level of consciousness, and skin condition.

An institution is responsible for defining how these monitoring parameters are to be collected through the development of policy and procedures. The policy and procedures should specify the type of equipment and physiologic data to be collected by the monitoring RN to provide continuous assessment of oxygenation, ventilation, circulation, and level of consciousness for a patient receiving conscious sedation and analgesia medications. The JCAHO (1996) recommends that when a level of sedation may result in the loss of protective reflexes, the same standards used for anesthesia care should be provided. Therefore consideration should be given to the types of medications to be administered by the RN, the desired depth of sedation, appropriate patient acuity level for nurse-monitored sedation, and the types of procedures that allow for a predictable outcome. Also, the JCAHO recommends that institutional protocols be consistent with professional standards and recommendations. The sources providing professional standards on the role of nonanesthesia RNs administering conscious sedation and analgesia are obtained from the state board of nursing, professional associations, current literature, and the institution's continuous quality improvement data. The JCAHO (1996) requires protocols for the administration of sedation to address the following:

- Sufficient qualified personnel present to perform the procedure and to monitor the patient
- Appropriate equipment for care and resuscitation
- Appropriate monitoring of vital signs—heart and respiratory rates and oxygenation
- Documentation of care
- Monitoring of outcomes

It is important to remember that the same standard of care be applied to all patients regardless of the location. Once specific monitoring parameters have been determined, the collection of these monitoring parameters (i.e., respiratory rate, oxygen saturation, blood pressure, cardiac rate and rhythm, and level of consciousness) may vary from unit to unit, depending on available monitoring equipment and sedation level.

In no event should reliance on a monitor supersede the continuous observation of a dedicated monitoring RN whose sole responsibility is to monitor the patient. It is not advisable to assign the monitoring RN additional responsibilities that require him/her to leave the patient unattended (i.e., out the room) even for a brief period. This places the patient at potential risk. It is imperative that the patient be appropriately monitored during the procedure to ensure rapid identification and correction of any problem to prevent serious complications and a possible fatal outcome.

Pulse

Assessing the pulse provides a reflection of the overall condition of the heart and the vascular system. The RN may assess the pulse rate by palpating an artery. The radial artery, which is the most commonly used site for older children and adults, may be palpated by placing the first two fingers gently on the lateral palmar area of the wrist. Gentle pressure is applied until pulsation is felt, with the artery never fully occluded (i.e., to the point where no pulsation is felt). Other pulse sites are described in Table 2-3. The apical pulse provides the most accurate assessment for children and adults with known dysrhythmias. To assess the apical pulse, place a stethoscope on the left side of the chest over the apex of the heart, between the fifth and sixth ribs at the midclavicular line. Count the pulse rate for a full 60 seconds.

Pulse Rate

The pulse should be evaluated for a period of at least 30 seconds. If the pulse is irregular, it should be assessed for a full 60 seconds. The pulse rate is initiated by the

TABLE 2-3 *Pulse Sites*

SITE	LOCATION	ASSESSMENT CRITERIA
Temporal	Over temporal bone of the head, above and lateral to the eye	Easily accessible site to assess pulse in children
Carotid	Along medial edge of sternocleidomastoid muscle in neck	Easily accessible site to assess character of peripheral pulse; used during physiologic shock or cardiac arrest when other sites are not palpable
Apical	Fourth to fifth intercostal space at midclavicular line	Site for auscultation of heart sounds
Brachial	Groove between biceps and triceps muscles at the antecubital fossa	Assesses status of circulation to lower arm Site used to auscultate blood pressure
Radial	Radial (thumb) side of forearm at the wrist	Common site to assess character of peripheral pulse; assesses status of circulation to hand
Ulnar	Ulnar side of forearm at the wrist	Assesses status of circulation to ulnar side of hand; used to assess an Allen test
Femoral	Below the inguinal ligament, midway between symphyis pubis and anterior superior iliac spine	Assesses character of pulse during physiologic shock or cardiac arrest when other pulses are not palpable; assesses status of circulation to the leg
Popliteal	Behind the knee in popliteal fossa	Assesses status of circulation to the lower leg
Posterior tibial	Inner side of each ankle, below medial malleolus	Assesses status of circulation to the foot
Dorsalis pedis	Along top of foot between extension tendons of great and first toe	Assesses status of circulation to the foot

From Perry, A. G., Potter, P. A. (1994). *Clinical nursing skills and techniques* (3rd ed.). St. Louis: Mosby.

sinoatrial node, which is located in the right atrium. Normal resting pulse for the adult is 60 to 100 beats per minute. If the pulse is less than 50 beats per minute, it is bradycardic. If the pulse is greater than 100 beats per minute, it is tachycardic. A variety of factors influence the pulse rate. Any heart rate falling below 50 beats per minute should be evaluated. For well-conditioned athletes, many of whom tolerate a rate less than 50 beats per minute without symptoms, no treatment is necessary. However, treatment is indicated if the patient is bradycardic and experiencing symptoms such as chest pain, dizziness, or dyspnea.

Most patients experience fear and anxiety about the impending procedure. This may result in sympathetic stimulation, which increases the pulse rate. Other factors that may cause tachycardia include hyperthyroidism, anemia, hypovolemia, and hypoxia. Also, tachycardia may be related to an increase in oxygen demand (e.g., hypoxemia). When it is suspected that the heart is trying to compensate for the increased demand by increasing the pulse, the cause should be determined.

Medications such as sympathomimetic drugs and beta blockers cause the pulse rate to speed up or slow down, respectively. It is important to know what current medications are being taken by the patient. Pulse rates also follow a person's circadian rhythm, with rates being slightly higher in the late afternoon.

Pulse Rhythm

Pulse rhythm should be assessed to determine if it is regular or irregular. A regular rhythm has pulsations occurring at regular intervals. A rhythm in which the pulse intervals are unevenly spaced is irregular and indicates a disturbance. An irregular rhythm is commonly referred to as a dysrhythmia or arrhythmia. The two terms are used interchangeably, with both indicating a disturbance in the normal rhythm. Through palpation the only determination that can be made is whether the pulse is regular or irregular. If an irregular rhythm is present, a 12-lead ECG may be ordered by the physician to confirm the dysrhythmia. The most frequent dysrhythmias are premature ventricular contractions and premature atrial contractions.

Pulse Quality

Palpation of the pulse allows assessment of the quality or strength of the pulse. The strength of the pulse can be rated on a scale from 0 to 4 (Table 2-4). The pulse feels stronger in the upper extremities than in the lower extremities. If during the procedure the pulse becomes weak, the patient should be assessed for hypovolemia or hypotension. If the pulse suddenly becomes very strong and bounding, the patient may be hypervolemic or hypertensive or may be experiencing sudden anxiety or pain related to the procedure.

A strong pulse followed by a weak one may indicate pulsus alternans and indicates further patient assessment. A characteristic of pulsus alternans is the palpation

TABLE 2-4 *Grading of Pulses*

GRADE	DESCRIPTION
0	Not palpable
+1	Difficult to palpate, thready, weak, easily obliterated with pressure
+2	Difficult to palpate; may be obliterated with pressure
+3	Easy to palpate; not easily obliterated with pressure
+4	Strong, bounding; not obliterated with pressure

From Wong, D. L. (1995). *Pediatric quick reference* (2nd. ed., p.1). St. Louis: Mosby. Reprinted with permission.

of alternate strong and weak beats usually caused by left-sided heart failure, severe hypertension, and coronary artery disease. The patient should be assessed to determine the potential risks for a procedure with the administration of conscious sedation and analgesia agents by a nonanesthesia provider.

Pulse Oximeter

One of the most common and most valuable monitoring devices used to assess oxygenation in a patient receiving conscious sedation and analgesia is the pulse oximeter. This instrument provides a noninvasive measure of the arterial hemoglobin oxygen saturation and pulse rate. Pulse oximeters are portable, easy to use, and may be run by battery, which allows for ease in transporting the patient while providing continuous uninterrupted monitoring. Knowledge of the principles of oxygen transport assists the nurse to interpret data from the pulse oximeter.

Oxygen is highly bound to hemoglobin. A single hemoglobin molecule may bind with zero to four molecules of oxygen (Wesmiller & Hoffman, 1989). A hemoglobin molecule that is 100% saturated contains four oxygen molecules; 75% saturated, three oxygen molecules; 50% saturated, two molecules; and 25% saturated, only one. Assessing the hemoglobin oxygen saturation (SaO_2), which is the ratio of saturated hemoglobin compared to the total hemoglobin molecules, gives the nurse a fairly accurate reflection of arterial oxygenation status.

Oxygen saturation (SaO_2) occurs in direct relation to the partial pressure of oxygen (PaO_2), as shown in the oxyhemoglobin dissociation curve (Figure 2-2). PaO_2 is the amount of oxygen that is dissolved in the blood. The normal range of PaO_2 is 80 to 100 mm Hg provided that the pH and the body temperature are normal. This is equivalent to an SaO_2 of 95% to 100%. The curve shifts when changes occur in body temperature, partial pressure of carbon dioxide (PCO_2), and hydrogen ion concentration (H^+). A decrease in body temperature, H^+, and PCO_2 results in the curve shifting to the right. This means that the oxygen attached to the hemoglobin is more easily released into the tissues. An increase in body temperature, H^+, and PCO_2 results

Describes relationship between Pao$_2$ (arterial oxygen tension) and Sao$_2$ (arterial hemoglobin oxygen saturation).

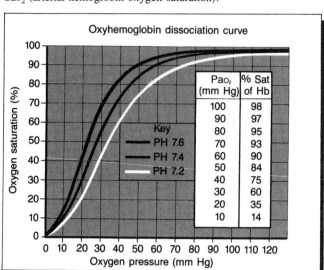

FIGURE 2-2 | Oxyhemoglobin dissociation curve. (From Wong, D.L. [1995]. *Pediatric quick reference* [2nd ed., p. 5.], St. Louis: Mosby. Reprinted with permission.)

Changes in the affinity of hemoglobin for oxygen shift the position of the oxyhemoglobin dissociation curve.

Standard curve (middle curve above): Assumes normal pH (7.4), temperature, Pco$_2$, and 2,3-DPG levels

Shift to left (upper curve above): Increases O$_2$ affinity of Hb: increased pH; decreased temperature, Pco$_2$, and 2,3-DPG

Shift to right (lower curve above): Decreases O$_2$ affinity of Hb: decreased pH; increased temperature, Pco$_2$, and 2,3-DPG

in a shift to the left. This means that the oxygen is binding more tightly to the hemoglobin, resulting in less oxygen available to oxygenate tissue.

The use of pulse oximetry has become a standard of care for the patient receiving conscious sedation and analgesia for the single reason that it provides a reliable indication of Sao$_2$. The monitoring RN should be proficient in interpreting readings from the pulse oximeter. If a saturation level falls below 95% but remains continuous, the patient's ventilation and oxygenation status should immediately be assessed, should be administered as appropriate, and the physician should be notified. Because of reports of up to a 2% margin of error in comparisons of invasive and noninvasive Sao$_2$ levels, arterial blood gases should be drawn for any rate that falls below 80% and remains continuous (Wesmiller & Hoffman, 1989).

The pulse oximeter includes a sensing device that contains a light-emitting diode and a photodetector. The transducer is placed over the ear lobe, fingertip, or nose. Wavelengths of light are passed through the vascular bed, and the amount of light that passes through is measured. Any patient movement may affect the reading and result in the sounding of an alarm.

Pulse oximetry provides an early indication of developing hypoxemia. It is an excellent device to assist the RN in monitoring the patient receiving conscious sedation and analgesia. Often the draping, positioning for a procedure, or room lighting makes it nearly impossible to observe the patient's ventilatory status. The use of pulse oximetry offers an added measure of providing continuous uninterrupted monitoring of the patient's arterial oxygenation status.

Respiration

Respiratory assessment should include the patient's past or current respiratory problems and smoking history. The RN should assess the rate, depth, and quality of respirations by inspection, palpation, percussion, and auscultation.

Inspection

The color of the patient's lips, oral mucosa, nail beds, and extremities should be assessed to determine the presence of cyanosis or pallor. The patient should be observed for signs of labored breathing such a nasal flaring. Children and males generally are diaphragmatic breathers; observation of abdominal movement is helpful in assessment of rate, depth, and quality. Females tend to move the entire thoracic cage with each breath.

The normal respiratory rate for the adult is between 12 and 20 breaths per minute, with pediatric rates varying by age (Table 2-5). Fewer than 12 breaths per

TABLE 2-5 *Normal Respirations and Heart Rates for Pediatric Patient*

AGE	RESPIRATION (BREATHS/MIN)	HEART (BEATS/MIN)
Infant (birth-12 mo)	30-60	120-160
Toddler (1-3 yr)	25-40	90-140
Preschool-age child (4-6 yr)	22-34	80-110
School-age child (6-12 yr)	18-30	75-100
Adolescent (13-18 yr)	12-20	60-100

From Meeker, M. H., & Rothrock, J. C. (1995). *Alexander's care of the patient in surgery* (10th ed., p. 1229). St. Louis: Mosby.

minute are considered bradypneic, and such a patient should be closely assessed. If conscious sedation and analgesia medications have been administered, oversedation should be ruled out as the cause. More than 20 breaths per minute are considered tachypneic and are most often related to preprocedure anxiety. Respirations should always be counted for one full minute.

Palpation

Following inspection, the patient's chest should be palpated to determine any obvious abnormalities. Respiratory expansion should be assessed by palpating bony structures of the chest. The practitioner's hands are placed over the lower posterior chest wall, and the patient is directed to take a few deep breaths. The assessment of equal lung expansion should be determined. The temperature, moisture, and turgor of the skin should be assessed.

Percussion

The monitoring nurse may percuss the patient's chest by placing the middle finger of one hand (i.e., pleximeter) flat against the chest wall and gently striking the distal portion of the middle finger with the middle finger of the other hand. This causes vibrations that the RN may hear and feel. Resonance is a low-pitched, hollow sound that is heard over the normal lung.

Auscultation

The monitoring RN should listen to the respirations. The patient with normal respirations breathes quietly and without difficulty. Abnormal breath sounds such as rales, rhonchi, or wheezing indicate a respiratory problem and should be thoroughly assessed to determine etiology and possible contraindications to nurse-monitored sedation because the sedatives-anxiolytics and narcotic analgesics administered for conscious sedation and analgesia have the potential to depress respirations and result in loss of protective reflexes.

Bilateral lung fields are auscultated with a stethoscope. The patient is directed to breathe deeply. A systematic approach should be used to auscultate the anterior, lateral, and posterior chest walls while comparing both sides.

Assessment of the respiratory system allows the monitoring RN to rule out any possible problems related to the administration of medications that may depress the respiratory system. It is essential to provide continuous uninterrupted monitoring of the respiratory status throughout the entire period of the patient's sedated state. Because of varying degrees of respiratory depression that occur as a result of medications administered, oxygen and oxygen delivery devices should be immediately available. Dyspnea or difficulty in breathing may be exhibited by sudden shallow respirations, nasal flaring, mouth breathing, combativeness, increasing anxiety level, and inability to cooperate during the procedure. Any of these symptoms should be reported to the physician immediately. The etiology (e.g., oversedation, undersedation, pain, idiosyncratic reaction) needs to be determined as soon as possible.

Blood Pressure

The monitoring RN should employ noninvasive methods for measuring the arterial blood pressure by using an aneroid or mercury type of sphygmomanometer or automated electronic monitor.

Manual Method

This method involves using a stethoscope and a sphygmomanometer with an inflatable blood pressure cuff. The cuff bladder width should be approximately 40% of the upper arm circumference. The length of the cuff bladder should be approximately 80% of the arm circumference. A cuff that is too narrow to too loose provides a falsely elevated blood pressure reading.

The most common placement of the blood pressure cuff is over the brachial artery. The lower edge of the cuff is positioned approximately 1 inch above the antecubital fossa, allowing the patient to slightly flex the elbow. The cuff is applied snugly, allowing two fingers to be easily inserted at the edge. The stethoscope is located and placed over the brachial artery. The blood pressure cuff is gently inflated to about 30 mm Hg above the point at which pulsations from the radial pulse disappear. The cuff is slowly deflated (2 to 3 mm Hg per second). The first sound heard is the systolic pressure. The cuff should continue to be deflated slowly to zero. The diastolic blood pressure is the disappearance point, where no sounds are heard.

Common errors

Incorrect application. The most common problem of applying a blood pressure cuff is incorrect position and improper size of the blood pressure cuff. Cuffs that are too short, too long, or too loose may result in an erroneous reading.

Obese arm. If an appropriate-size cuff is not available for the upper arm, an appropriate-size cuff for the forearm may be applied. The same technique as previously described should be used, with a stethoscope placed over the radial artery at the wrist to ascultate systolic and diastolic pressures.

Anxious patient. The most common cause of a high blood pressure reading is anxiety related to the impending procedure. The patient should be allowed time to become relaxed and comfortable before another reading is taken.

Auscultatory gap. A gap that results in the loss of sound between the systolic and diastolic pressures is commonly noted in patients with high blood pressure. Although no sound can be heard, the pulse will be present. It is important for the nurse to palpate the radial pulse and inflate the pressure approximately 30 mm Hg above the point where no pulsations are felt. Otherwise, a false low reading may be obtained.

Automatic Method

Arterial blood pressure monitoring of the patient receiving conscious sedation and analgesia is commonly monitored by an oscillometric device. This monitoring device allows for blood pressure readings to be taken at specified intervals. In addition to blood pressure, readings of mean arterial pressure and heart rate are displayed on most models. The cuff contains an actuator and transducer for detection of arterial wall oscillations. The cuff is applied with the same guidelines used as for the conventional method.

Electrocardiogram

The RN responsible for the management of care for the patient receiving conscious sedation and analgesia should have a basic knowledge and understanding of cardiac monitoring and dysrhythmia interpretation. An electrocardiograph continuously monitors the heart rate and rhythm and detects cardiac dysrhythmias. The use of an electrocardiograph is not considered a universal standard for monitoring the patient receiving conscious sedation and analgesia. In fact, some units monitor heart rate and rhythm by the simple method of palpation, or they use a pulse oximeter monitor to detect dysrhythmias.

Although various types of cardiac monitors are on the market, most contain an easy-to-locate on-off switch, oscilloscope, brightness control, heart rate display, rate alarms, position control, size control, gain control, mm/sec control, run/hold/freeze control, calibration control, mode control, and lead control. Lead II is commonly selected to monitor the heart's electrical activity because monitoring in lead II is useful in assessing P waves, PR intervals, and atrial dysrhythmias (Figure 2-3). When an electrocardiograph is used for monitoring, it is important to remember:

1. A prominent P wave represents atrial activity and should be displayed on the ECG. Leads that easily identify the P wave should be selected.
2. The QRS amplitude should be high enough to trigger the ratemeter.
3. Monitoring with an electrocardiograph identifies only disturbances in rhythms. If more elaborate ECG interpretation is indicated, a complete 12-lead ECG should be ordered by the physician.
4. Attention should be given to artifact. Because artifact may appear as a wavy baseline resembling ventricular fibrillation, the clinical status of the patient should always be assessed first.

Capnography

Monitoring expired carbon dioxide concentrations is increasingly being used by the RN for monitoring the patient receiving deep sedation. A nasal adapter set is inserted into a nasal prong used for oxygen administration. This allows for monitoring end-expiratory carbon dioxide. Capnography is used for early detection of hy-

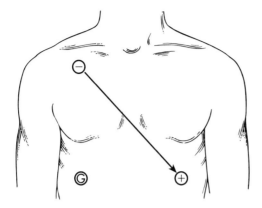

FIGURE 2-3 | Monitoring in lead II.

poventilation and airway obstruction. False readings may occur if the patient is a mouth breather or the unit becomes displaced.

Level of Consciousness

The monitoring RN who administers conscious sedation and analgesia medications should titrate the medications in small increments until the desired sedative level is achieved. The optimal sedative level is one in which all the patient's protective reflexes are intact. The patient should be relaxed, easily aroused from sleep, and able to respond to verbal communication and commands.

The Ramsay Sedation Scale (Ramsay et al., 1974) is frequently used in intensive care units, but it is limited in clinical application to assessment of a patient's level of consciousness. Although critics argue the application of the Ramsay Sedation Scale in the intensive care unit (Hansen-Flaschen et al., 1994), its use may be appropriate in areas where conscious sedation and analgesia medications are administered during short-term therapeutic, diagnostic, or surgical procedures. With the scale used as a guide, the medications administered are titrated to the desired level of sedation requested by the physician (Box 2-2). A patient profile for each level might suggest the following:

- Ramsay Sedation Scale 1 = Patient is admitted to the preprocedure area experiencing anxiety and fear regarding the impending procedure.
- Ramsay Sedation Scale 2 = Patient is alert, talkative, cooperative, calm, and relaxed during the procedure.
- Ramsay Sedation Scale 3 = Patient is cooperative, calm, and relaxed with eyes closed. Patient responds to verbal command.
- Ramsay Sedation Scale 4 = Patient is asleep. Patient is quick to respond to a light tap between the eyebrows or to calling of his/her name loudly.

| BOX | 2-2 *Ramsay Sedation Scale* |

LEVEL OF SEDATION: CONSCIOUS

1 = Patient is anxious and agitated or restless or both.

2 = Patient is cooperative, oriented, and tranquil.

3 = Patient responds to commands only.

LEVEL OF SEDATION: DEEP

4 = Patient exhibits brisk response to light glabellar tap or loud auditory stimulus.

5 = Patient exhibits a sluggish response to light glabellar tap or loud response.

6 = Patient exhibits no response.

From Ramsey, M. A. E., Savage, T. M., Simpson, B. R. J., & Goodwin, R. (1974). Controlled sedation with alphaxalone-alphadolone. *British Medical Journal, 2,* 656-659.

- Ramsay Sedation Scale 5 = Patient is asleep and more heavily sedated. Patient is slow to respond to a light tap between the eyebrows or to loud calling of name. Stimuli may need to be repeated before patient responds.
- Ramsay Sedation Scale 6 = Patient is unresponsive. This level of sedation is beyond the intent and scope of practice for the RN administering conscious sedation and analgesia during short-term therapeutic or diagnostic procedures.

The Conscious Sedation Scale (Table 2-6) is another tool for objective assessment of the patient receiving conscious sedation and analgesia; it is also a documentation tool (Clark, 1994). The Conscious Sedation Scale allows for monitoring and scoring of the patient's (1) emotional affect, (2) level of consciousness, (3) physical reaction to discomfort or pain, (4) variation in vital signs, and (5) degree of amnesia. The patient is given a grade of 0 to 2; an overall score of 8 to 10 reflects an optimally sedated patient.

Implementation of both of these tools provides a more objective assessment of the patient receiving conscious sedation and analgesia. If these tools are used in an institution, both RNs and physicians should be familiar and understand the application and limitation of each one. Understanding the various levels and patient profiles on the conscious sedation and analgesia continuum is key to achieving a standard of administration that is consistent among the various units and disciplines.

POSTPROCEDURE ASSESSMENT

Because the patient has not received general anesthesia, he or she will most likely be transferred to a phase II level of care. The patient may go directly to an ambulatory care unit, a medical-surgical floor, or a recovery room in the unit where the procedure

TABLE 2-6 *Conscious Sedation Scale*

OPTIMAL RANGE: 8-10	GRADE		
PARAMETER (CIRCLE ONE)	0	1	2
Emotional affect 0 1 2 _____	1. Flat affect 2. Does not respond to commands or stimuli	1. Anxious or uneasy (>50%) 2. Does not respond to commands appropriately	1. Quiescent, tranquil (>75%) 2. Responds to commands appropriately
Level of consciousness 0 1 2 _____	1. Unarousable/stuporus 2. Protective reflexes absent	1. Intermittent arousal or awake/aware 2. Protective reflexes present	1. Drowsy or asleep, easily arousable 2. Protective reflexes present
Physical reaction to discomfort or pain 0 1 2 _____	1. Flaccid/non-responsive 2. No exhibition or c/o discomfort or pain	1. Restless and/or resistive 2. Vocalization throughout majority of procedure (>50%)	1. Generally at ease/rest 2. May occasionally exhibit symptoms or vocalize c/o discomfort/pain
Variation in vital signs 0 1 2 _____	1. Respiratory depression and/or decrease in cardiovascular function 2. Intervention necessary	1. No beneficial change in respiratory or cardiovascular function	1. Therapeutic alteration in respiratory/cardio-vascular function 2. No intervention necessary
Degree of amnesia 0 1 2 _____	1. Total amnesia (secondary to stuporous condition and loss of protective reflexes)	1. Recall of 75%-100% of procedure	1. Minimal recall (<25%) or total amnesia

CSS Score _____ Comments:

was conducted. If the patient is transported to another area, a verbal report should be given by the monitoring RN to the receiving nurse or caregiver. It is important for the monitoring RN to report the patient's name, procedure, medical problems, dosage, time of last medication(s) administered for conscious sedation and analgesia, and any adverse reactions. Recovery time depends on the type of medication(s) administered, dose, time of administration, and patient's level of consciousness.

The same monitoring parameters are applicable during the recovery phase that were used during the procedure. These include assessment of the respiratory rate, oxygen saturation, blood pressure, cardiac rate and rhythm, level of consciousness, and skin condition. In addition, if appropriate, the patient should be monitored for operative site bleeding, nausea and vomiting, and appropriate pain management.

The patient receiving conscious sedation and analgesia is discharged when the criteria that have been determined by the physician are met. Although there is no standard set of criteria that must be met for the patient receiving conscious sedation and analgesia, typically the criteria include stable vital signs; stable respiratory status; level of consciousness; orientation to person, place, and time; ability to dress with minimal assistance; ability to walk without assistance; controlled nausea/vomiting; minimal discomfort and pain; an understanding of postoperative care; and a responsible adult escort available to care for the patient after discharge from the institution.

CONCLUSION

Every patient undergoing a short-term diagnostic, therapeutic, or surgical procedure under conscious sedation and analgesia deserves safe quality care regardless of the provider. The attitude of "It's only a local" has resulted in some patients receiving care that is far below the standard. Minimal monitoring parameters for the patient receiving conscious sedation and analgesia include continuous assessment of the respiratory rate, oxygen saturation, blood pressure, cardiac rate and rhythm, level of consciousness, and skin condition. This chapter has suggested a monitoring process for the patient that includes the following phases:

- Preprocedure Phase: Obtaining the baseline health information (e.g., vital signs, physical examination, medical and medication history).
- Intraprocedure Phase: Continuous monitoring of vital signs (e.g., heart rate and rhythm, respiratory rate, blood pressure), oxygenation (e.g., oxygen saturation, skin condition), and level of consciousness.
- Postprocedure Phase: Continuation of procedure monitoring parameters until the effects of conscious sedation and analgesia medications have decreased and the patient's level of consciousness is at the preprocedure state.

The intent of monitoring by a nonanesthesia provider is not to sacrifice quality by providing a lesser standard of care than the anesthesia provider but to provide the patient with a quality and standard of care to enhance patient safety to safeguard against an untoward outcome.

REFERENCES

American Society of Anesthesiologists. (1995). *Guidelines for sedation and analgesia by non-anesthesiologists.* Park Ridge, IL: Author.

Chrisman, B. B., Watson, M. A., & McDonald, D. E. (1988). Outpatient anesthesia. *Journal of Dermatology Surgical Oncology, 14*(9), 939-946.

Clark, B. (1994). A new approach to assessment and documentation of conscious sedation during endoscopic examinations. *Gastroenterology Nursing, 16* (5), 199-203.

Cummins, R. O. (Ed.). (1994). *Textbook of advanced cardiac life support.* Dallas: American Heart Association.

Dierdorf, S. F. (1995). ASA practice guidelines for management of the difficult airway. *Current Reviews for Nurse Anesthetists, 17*(17), 168-171.

Hansen-Flaschen, J., Cowen, J., & Polomano, R. (1994). Beyond the Ramsay scale: Need for a validated measure of sedating drug efficacy in the intensive care unit. *Critical Care Medicine, 22*(5), 732-733.

Joint Commission on Accreditation of Health Care Organizations (JCAHO). (1996). Comprehensive accreditation manual for hospitals. Oakbrook Terrace, IL: Author.

Malamed, S. F. (1995). *Sedation: a guide to patient management* (3rd ed.). St. Louis: Mosby.

Ramsay, M., Savege, T., Simpson, B., & Goodwin, R. (1974). Controlled sedation with alphaxalone-alphadolone. *British Medical Journal, 2,* 656-659.

Smith, C. R., & Petty, B. G. (1988). Specific complications of medical management. In A. M. Harvey, R. J. Johns, V. A. McKusick, A. H. Owens, & R. S. Ross (Eds.), *The principles and practice of medicine* (22nd ed.). Norwalk, CT: Appleton & Lange.

Wesmiller, S. W., Hoffman, L. A. (1989). Interpreting your patient's oxygenation status. *Orthopaedic Nursing 8*(6), 56-60.

BIBLIOGRAPHY

Comer, D. M. (1992). Pulse oximetry: Implications for practice. *Journal of Obstetric, Gynecologic, & Neonatal Nursing,* 21(1), 35-41.

Eichhorn, J. H. (1989). Prevention of intraoperative anesthesia accidents and related severe injury through safety monitoring. *Anesthesiology, 70,* 572-577.

Fleischer, D. (1989). Monitoring the patient receiving conscious sedation for gastrointestinal endoscopy. *Gastrointestinal Endoscopy, 35,* 265, 267.

Fleischer, D. (1990). Monitoring for conscious sedation: Perspective of the gastrointestinal endoscopist. *Gastrointestinal Endoscopy, 36*(3), S19-22.

Henneman, E. A., & Henneman, P. L. (1989). Intricacies of blood pressure measurement: Reexamining the rituals. *Heart Lung, 18*(3), 263-273.

Holzman, R. S., Cullen, D. J., Eichhorn, J. H., & Philip, J. H. (1994). Guidelines for sedation by non-anesthesiologists during diagnostic and therapeutic procedures. *Journal of Clinical Anesthesia, 6,* 265-276.

Kidwell, J. A. (1991). Nursing care for the patient receiving conscious sedation during gastrointestinal endoscopic procedures. *Gastroenterology Nursing, 13,* 136-137.

Maree, S. M. (1992). Benzodiazepines and their reversal. *Current Reviews for Nurse Anesthetists, 15,* 53-60.

Murphy, E. (1988). Legal considerations in RN monitoring of intravenous sedation. *AORN Journal, 48*(6), 1184-1187.

Murphy, E. (1993). Monitoring IV conscious sedation, the legal scope of practice. *AORN Journal, 57*(2), 512-514.

O'Connor, K. W., Jones, S. (1990). Oxygen desaturation is common and clinically underappreciated during elective endoscopic procedures. *Gastrointestinal Endoscopy,* (Suppl 3), S2-4.

Sanders, A. (1989). End-tidal carbon dioxide monitoring during cardiopulmonary resuscitation: A prognostic indicator for survival. *JAMA, 262*(10), 1347-1351.

Skoog, R. E. (1989). Capnography in the post anesthesia care unit. *Journal of Post Anesthesia Nursing, 4*(3), 147-155.

Spry, C. C. (1990). Perioperative nurses should keep monitoring within their specialty. *AORN Journal, 51*(4), 1071-1072.

Spyr, J., & Preach, M. A. (1990). Pulse oximetry: understanding the concept, knowing the limits. *RN, 53*(5), 38-45.

Thilo, E. H., Anderson, D., Wasserstein, M. L., Schmidt, J., & Luckey, D. (1993). Saturation by pulse oximetry: Comparison of the results obtained by instruments of different brands. *Journal of Pediatrics, 122*(4), 620-626.

Watson, D. S., & James, D. (1990). Intravenous conscious sedation: Implications of monitoring patients receiving local anesthesia. *AORN Journal, 51*(6), 1512-1522.

Pharmacology

III

One of the main purposes of this book is to provide a resource for the nonanesthesia provider who is responsible for the management of conscious sedation and analgesia in the patient undergoing a short-term therapeutic, diagnostic, or surgical procedure. Proper management of conscious sedation and analgesia is directly related to patient satisfaction. To achieve adequate management, the monitoring registered nurse (RN) administers a variety of medications until the desired patient effects are achieved (e.g., slightly slurred speech, restful sleep, cooperation, no evidence of discomfort, stable vital signs). The spectrum of pain and anxiety control (Figure 3-1) illustrates various techniques that include pharmacologic and non-pharmacologic interventions. This chapter focuses on the administration of intravenous (IV) medications to achieve adequate conscious sedation and analgesia.

INTRAVENOUS ADMINISTRATION

Administration of medications through IV injection is characterized by rapid onset of action, approximately 20 to 30 seconds from the time the medication is administered until the desired patient effects are observed. IV injection provides a direct route of entry into the bloodstream. If administered incorrectly, it may have direct, adverse patient reactions (i.e., drop in blood pressure, respiratory depression, cardiac arrest).

Before any IV medication is administered, the RN should be knowledgeable about each medication—recommended dilution, recommended dose, adverse reactions, compatibility with other medications and solutions—and aware of any patient allergies.

IV Push

The technique of IV push is the administration of a medication directly into a vein through a secure IV catheter, generally located in a large peripheral vein. The dose and rate of administration should follow pharmaceutical recommendations and should not be exceeded. Usually no more than 1 mg over a 1-minute period is recommended (Shannon, Wilson, & Stang, 1995, p. 21). However, some medications have a high potency level and are administered in micrograms (μg), not milligrams. Therefore the RN should always check the recommended rate of administration for each drug.

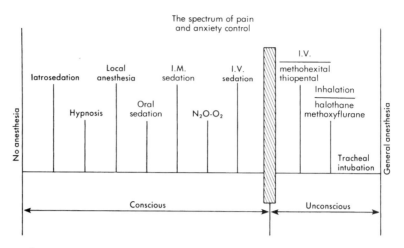

FIGURE 3-1 | Spectrum of pain and anxiety control. Illustration of various techniques available for patient management. Vertical bar represents loss of consciousness. (From Malamed, S. F. [1995]. *Sedation: A guide to patient management* [3rd ed.]. St. Louis: Mosby.)

IV Titration

This technique involves direct administration into a vein, with titration of small increments of the medication until the desired patient effects are achieved. Following pharmaceutical guidelines, the RN may dilute the medication with a compatible solution into a syringe and slowly administer it by pushing the syringe plunger, while observing for the desired patient effects and any adverse reactions.

IV Continuous Infusion

This technique is frequently used in an intensive care unit (ICU) for patients in need of continuous sedation and pain management. Opioids are frequently supplemented by the administration of a benzodiazepine. Medications are mixed according to pharmaceutical guidelines and administered through a controlled-infusion device at a fixed rate to achieve the desired patient effect.

IV Intermittent Infusion

This method is most commonly known as the IV piggyback method. The medication is mixed into a set solution and "piggybacked" into a continuous infusion of compatible solution already being administered to the patient. The intermittent infusion may be delivered through a controlled-infusion device and is used primarily for conscious sedation and pain management in ICUs.

BENZODIAZEPINES

General Pharmacology

In the mid-1950s work toward the development of a new tranquilizer produced unexpected results (Sternbach, 1978), that is, benzodiazepines with muscle relaxation, sedative, and anticonvulsant properties. Today benzodiazepines are widely administered to achieve a sedated state in which the patient may be amnesic while maintaining consciousness during a short-term therapeutic, diagnostic, or surgical procedure.

Commonly administered benzodiazepines include diazepam, lorazepam, and midazolam. Desirable pharmacologic characteristics include amnesia, increased seizure threshold to local anesthetic agents, minimal depression of respiratory system when titrated to individual response, minimal hemodynamic effects, and excellent sedative, muscle relaxation, and antianxiety properties.

Mechanism of Action

The mechanism of action for benzodiazepines appears to be related to highly dense receptors found in the olfactory bulb, cerebral cortex, cerebellum, hippocampus, substantia nigra, and inferior colliculus. Less dense benzodiazepine receptors are found in the striatum, lower brain stem, and spinal cord. The specific receptor sites are part of the gammaaminobutyric acid (GABA) complex. The administration of a benzodiazepine facilitates inhibitory actions of GABA, allowing for a greater amount of GABA to be present at the postsynaptic nerve endings. This action results in inhibiting certain pathways of the central nervous system (CNS), resulting in the anticonvulsant, sedation, muscle relaxation, and antianxiety properties. The benzodiazepine antagonist flumazenil blocks the central effects of benzodiazepines and is often administered to reverse the sedative and amnestic effects after procedures that use a benzodiazepine.

Pharmacokinetics

The three benzodiazepines used most often for conscious sedation and analgesia may be classified according to their biotransformation and half-life: short lasting—midazolam; intermediate lasting—lorazepam; and long lasting—diazepam. Diazepam and midazolam are metabolized by hepatic microsomal oxidation. This oxidation process may be decreased in the older adult, resulting in a longer duration of action because of a slower clearance of the benzodiazepine; both hepatic dysfunction and the administration of certain medications (e.g., cimetidine) may impair the oxidizing process. Lorazepam is metabolized by hepatic glucuronide conjugation. Glucuronide conjugation is less affected by advanced age and medications that impair the oxidizing process. Of the three benzodiazepines, diazepam is the only one that is broken down into active metabolites (i.e., oxazepam and desmethyldiazepam), resulting in a prolonged duration of action.

Clinical Use

The benzodiazepines are popular and are administered as a premedication, during a surgical procedure to achieve a state of conscious sedation and analgesia, as an induction agent for general anesthesia, during general anesthesia as part of the balanced anesthesia triad, and postoperatively.

The widespread use of benzodiazepines for conscious sedation and analgesia is due to the resulting desirable effects on the patient: amnesia, minimal variation on physiologic monitoring parameters, suppression of seizure activity, and a relaxed sedative state. Because all benzodiazepines may cause respiratory depression, the patient should be properly monitored and the nonanesthesia provider should have proficient skills to maintain an airway in the event of an emergency. IV administration of a benzodiazepine allows for titration to the desired level of sedation (Table 3-1).

The most popular and most widely administered of the three benzodiazepines discussed here is midazolam. Midazolam has a rapid onset, produces excellent amnesic effects, and has a shorter duration of action than diazepam or lorazepam. It is three to four times more potent than diazepam. Diazepam is the longest lasting and is generally not administered for short procedures. Lorazepam is most often administered for procedures that are expected to last at least 4 hours.

The effects of benzodiazepines may be reversed with the antagonist flumazenil. Flumazenil competes with the inhibitory action of the GABA benzodiazepine receptor sites. Since flumazenil is benzodiazepine specific, it does not reverse the analgesia effect of narcotic(s) administered for analgesia.

DIAZEPAM
(dye-AYZ-eh-pam)

TRADE NAMES: Diazemuls, Diazepam Intensol, Rival, Valium, Valrelease, Vivol, Zetran

CLASSIFICATION: Anticonvulsant, anxiolytic, benzodiazepine, CNS agent

TABLE 3-1 *Intravenous Benzodiazepines*

DRUG	RECOMMENDED DOSAGE (IV)	PEAK EFFECTS (MIN)	HALF-LIFE (HR)	DURATION OF ACTION (HR)
Diazepam	5-10 mg q 2-4 hr	10-15	20-80	2-4
Lorazepam	2-4 mg q 2-4 hr	15-20	10-20	6-8
Midazolam	2.5-5 mg q hr	3-5	1-12	1.5-2

NOTES: Diazepam was first synthesized in 1959. It was found to have excellent antianxiety, skeletal muscle relaxant, and anticonvulsant properties. During the 1960s it became one of the most widely prescribed medications in the United States. Today diazepam is a useful premedication and is occasionally administered to decrease anxiety and apprehension during a short-term therapeutic, diagnostic, or surgical procedure. Following IV administration the patient may experience anterograde amnesia, which is lack of recall for a brief period following the injection of a medication such as diazepam.

PHARMACOKINETICS: *Onset:* 30 to 60 minutes PO; 15 to 30 minutes IM; 1 to 5 minutes IV. *Peak:* 1 to 2 hours PO; 10 to 30 minutes IV. *Duration:* 2 to 6 hours. *Metabolism:* Occurs in the liver by hepatic microsomal oxidation. The oxidation process may be impaired in patients with liver disease, advanced age, or coadministration of medications that inhibit microsomal oxidizing enzymes (e.g., cimetidine, isoniazid, and certain estrogens). Active metabolites include desmethyldiazepam and oxazepam, which account for prolonged effects of this medication. *Elimination:* Half-life is 20 to 40 hours (up to 80 hours in the older adult patient); excreted in urine.

CONTRAINDICATIONS AND PRECAUTIONS: Do not administer this drug in the presence of known hypersensitivity to diazepam. It may be administered to patients with acute narrow-angle glaucoma or open-angle glaucoma if that condition is medically managed. Because diazepam is metabolized in the liver and excreted by the kidneys, it should be administered with caution in patients with decreased liver or kidney function. Because phenothiazines, narcotics, barbiturates, monoamine oxidase (MAO) inhibitors, and antidepressants may potentiate diazepam's CNS effects, they should be administered cautiously.

ADVERSE REACTIONS: *CNS:* Drowsiness; confusion; depression; dysarthria; headache; hypoactivity; slurred speech; syncopy; tremor; vertigo. *GI:* Constipation; nausea. *GU:* Incontinence; changes in libido; urinary retention. *CV:* Bradycardia; cardiovascular collapse; hypotension. *EENT:* Blurred vision; diplopia; nystagmus. *Skin:* Urticaria; skin rash. *Other:* Hiccups; changes in salivation; neutropenia; jaundice.

DOSAGE AND ADMINISTRATION
Premedication
Adult: PO: 2 to 10 mg. *IM:* Inject 5 to 10 mg deeply into the muscle approximately 30 minutes before the procedure.

INTRAVENOUS CONSCIOUS SEDATION
Adult: IV: Slowly titrate diazepam until the initiation of slurred speech. Initial titration generally does not exceed 10 mg. Administer slowly over 1 minute for each

5 mg injected. If the patient has not received any premedication, up to 20 mg may be necessary to achieve the desired level of sedation necessary. If diazepam is administered with a narcotic, decrease the dose of the narcotic by one third and titrate in small increments to achieve the desired effect.

CONTINUOUS INFUSION (DOUCET ET AL., 1995)

Adult: 2 to 4 mg/hr (range, 1 to 15 mg/hr), with a recommended dilution of 20 mg of diazepam in 500 ml of D_5W (0.04 mg/ml; maximum concentration, 0.1 mg/ml); administer through a controlled-infusion device; maximum daily dose, 360 mg.

NURSING CONSIDERATIONS

Assessment

- Assess for medications known to inhibit the activity of microsomal oxidizing enzymes (e.g., cimetidine, isoniazid).
- Assess for medications known to intensify the CNS effect when administered with diazepam: for example, phenothiazines, narcotics, barbiturates, MAO inhibitors, and antidepressants.
- Assess for any abnormalities in liver and kidney function.
- Assess respiratory rate, oxygen saturation, blood pressure, cardiac rate and rhythm, level of consciousness, and skin condition.

Intervention

- Do not administer into small veins (e.g., dorsum of hand or wrist).
- Inject slowly through an infusing IV line over 1 minute for each 5 mg.
- It is not recommended that diazepam be mixed or diluted with other solutions; if administered IV, the drug should be administered directly into the vein or at a port as close to the vein as possible.
- Administer IM injection into deep muscle mass.
- Avoid intraarterial administration.
- Have suction equipment and a positive-pressure breathing device, oxygen, and appropriate airways in the room where diazepam is to be administered intravenously for conscious sedation and analgesia.
- Have an emergency cart immediately accessible.
- Administer cautiously to the older adults, debilitated patients, or those with cardiopulmonary disease.
- The nonanesthesia provider administering diazepam should be skilled at supporting a patient's oxygenation and ventilation status.

Desired Outcome

- Patient has decrease in anxiety and apprehension during procedure.

LORAZEPAM
(lor-AZE-pam)

TRADE NAME: Ativan

CLASSIFICATION: Anxiolytic, benzodiazepine, CNS agent, sedative-hypnotic

NOTES: Lorazepam (Ativan) is a benzodiazepine that is occasionally administered for its sedative effects (i.e., sleepiness, drowsiness, amnesia) during a procedure that is anticipated to last more than 2 hours. The intended sedative effects last 6 to 8 hours and significantly limit its use for outpatient procedures.

PHARMACOKINETICS: Biotransformation of lorazepam occurs in the liver via a process called conjugation. Conjugation is a principal pathway and is less susceptible to factors such as age, liver impairment, and drugs that inhibit microsomal oxidizing enzymes (e.g., cimetidine). *Onset:* 60 to 120 seconds IV; 15 to 30 minutes IM. *Peak:* 60 to 90 minutes IM. *Metabolism:* Occurs in the liver by the principal pathway of glucuronide conjugation. *Duration:* 6 to 8 hours. *Elimination:* Half-life is 16 hours IM and IV; excreted in urine.

CONTRAINDICATIONS AND PRECAUTIONS: Clinical trials reported that patients older than 50 years may experience more profound and prolonged effects from IV administration. Because of the risk of underventilation and apnea, this drug should be administered with caution in older adults, very ill patients, or patients with limited pulmonary reserve. It is contraindicated for use in patients with known hypersensitivity to benzodiazepines or with acute narrow-angle glaucoma.

ADVERSE REACTIONS: *CNS:* Excessive sleepiness and drowsiness; hallucinations; dizziness. *CV:* Hypertension or hypotension. *Ear:* Depressed hearing. *Eye:* Diplopia; blurred vision. *GI:* Nausea and vomiting. *Respiratory:* Partial airway obstruction. *Skin:* Rash.

DOSAGE AND ADMINISTRATION
Premedication
Adult (IM): 2 to 4 mg (0.05 mg/kg) 2 hours before procedure.

Intravenous Conscious Sedation
Adult (IV): 0.044 mg/kg or up to 2 mg 15 to 20 minutes before procedure.

Continuous Infusion (Doucet et al., 1995)
Dilute 20 mg in 200 ml of solution (e.g., sterile water for injection, 0.9% sodium chloride, D_5W); administer at 0.5 mg to 2 mg/hr; maximum concentration 1 mg/10 ml of solution.

NURSING CONSIDERATIONS
Assessment

- Assess for medications known to intensify the CNS effect when administered with lorazepam: phenothiazines, narcotics, barbiturates, MAO inhibitors, and antidepressants.
- Assess for any abnormalities in liver and kidney function.
- Assess respiratory rate, oxygen saturation, blood pressure, cardiac rate and rhythm, level of consciousness, and skin condition.

Intervention

- For IV administration, dilute medication with equal amounts of compatible solution (e.g., sterile water for injection, sodium chloride injection, or 5% dextrose injection). Dilution is not recommended for IM injection.
- Inject slowly through an infusing IV line or directly into vein. The rate should not exceed 2 mg per minute.
- Administer IM undiluted injection into deep muscle mass.
- Avoid intraarterial administration.
- Have suction and a positive-pressure breathing device, oxygen, and appropriate airways in the room where lorazepam is to be administered.
- Have an emergency cart immediately accessible.
- The RN administering lorazepam should be skilled at supporting a patient's oxygenation and ventilation status.

Desired Outcome

- Patient has decrease in anxiety and apprehension during procedure.
- Patient has diminished recall of events during procedure.

MIDAZOLAM HYDROCHLORIDE
(my-DAYZ-oh-lam)

TRADE NAME: Versed

CLASSIFICATION: Anxiolytic, benzodiazepine, CNS agent, general anesthetic, sedative-hypnotic

NOTES: Midazolam was first introduced to the U.S. market in 1986. Since that time it has rapidly replaced diazepam for the administration of conscious sedation and analgesia. Midazolam has a rapid onset of action and a short elimination half-life and produces excellent amnestic effects. Midazolam is metabolized in the liver into two nonactive metabolites and is excreted in the urine. It is water soluble with a low incidence of venous irritation and injection site discomfort.

PHARMACOKINETICS: *Onset:* 15 minutes IM; 30 to 60 seconds IV. *Peak:* 30 to 60 minutes IM; 10 to 15 minutes IV. *Duration:* 1 to 2.5 hours IV. *Elimination:* Half-life is 1.2 to 12.3 hours IV; excreted in urine.

CONTRAINDICATIONS AND PRECAUTIONS: Contraindicated for patients with known hypersensitivity to midazolam or acute narrow-angle glaucoma. This drug may be administered to patients with open-angle glaucoma, if receiving medical therapy. It is not recommended for use during pregnancy or in obstetrics. From clinical studies guidelines for pediatric administration have been developed. This drug should be administered cautiously in older patients and those with chronic disease or decreased pulmonary reserve.

ADVERSE REACTIONS: Clinical trials for the investigation of midazolam use included the following findings: fluctuations in vital signs following parenteral administration included decreased tidal volume and/or decreased respiratory rate in 23.3% of patients following IV administration and in 10.8% of patients following IM administration. Apnea was reported in 15.4% of patients after IV administration, as well as variations in blood pressure and pulse rate.

The following additional adverse reaction was reported after IM administration: headache (1.3%). At the IM injection site the following reactions were reported: pain (3.7%), induration (0.5%), redness (0.5%), and muscle stiffness (0.3%).

The following additional reactions were reported subsequent to IV administration: hiccups (3.9%), nausea (2.8%), vomiting (2.6%), coughing (1.3%), oversedation (1.6%), headache (1.5%), drowsiness (1.2%). At the IV site the following reactions were reported: tenderness (5.6%), pain during injection (5.0%), redness (2.6%), induration (1.7%), or phlebitis (0.4%).

Other adverse reactions that were observed following IV administration and occurring at an incidence less than 1.0% include the following: *CNS:* Retrograde amnesia; euphoria; confusion; argumentativeness; nervousness; anxiety; grogginess; restlessness; emergence delirium or agitation; prolonged emergence from anesthesia; dreaming during emergence; sleep disturbance, insomnia; nightmares; athetoid movements; ataxia; dizziness; dysphoria; slurred speech; dysphonia; paresthesia. *CV:* Bigeminy; premature ventricular contractions; vasovagal episode; tachycardia; nodal rhythm. *GI:* Acid taste; excessive salivation; retching. *Skin:* Hives; hivelike elevation at injection site; swelling or feeling of burning, warmth, or coldness at injection site; rash; pruritus. *Respiratory:* Laryngospasm; bronchospasm; dyspnea; hyperventilation; sneezing; shallow respirations; airway obstruction; tachypnea. *Other:* Yawning; lethargy; chills; weakness; toothache; faint feeling; hematoma.

DOSAGE AND ADMINISTRATION
Premedication

Adult: IM: 0.07 to 0.08 mg/kg (average dose is 5 mg); administer 1 hour before procedure.

Intravenous Conscious Sedation

Healthy adults younger than age 60 years: Slowly titrate 1.0 to 2.5 mg until the initiation of slurred speech. Initial titration should not exceed 2.5 mg of midazolam. Administer over at least a 2-minute period. Never administer by rapid or single bolus. If additional medication is indicated, titrate in small increments (e.g., 0.5 mg) and wait an additional 2 minutes to evaluate the sedative effect. If opioids or other CNS depressants have been administered as a premedication, the patient will require about 30% less midazolam than would an unpremedicated patient.

Patients older than 60 years, debilitated, or chronically ill: Older adults and those with chronic disease or decreased pulmonary reserve are at increased risk for hypoventilation or apnea. Therefore titrate in smaller increments and at a slower rate (e.g., 1 mg or less every 30 to 45 seconds). If additional titration is necessary, administer no more than 1 mg over 2 minutes. Wait an additional 2 minutes after each increment to evaluate patient effect. Usually no more than 3.5 mg is necessary. Patients in these categories who have been premedicated with an opioid or other CNS depressant require about 50% less midazolam.

Maintenance Dose

If during the procedure additional doses are necessary to maintain the desired level of sedation, slowly titrate midazolam in small increments to desired effects (i.e., 25% of the initial dose administered to achieve the desired level of sedation).

Continuous Infusion

Loading dose of 0.01 to 0.05 mg/kg (0.5-4 mg for typical adult), followed by maintenance infusion of 0.02 to 0.1 mg/kg/hr (1-7 mg/hr), must be via infusion pump.

NURSING CONSIDERATIONS
Assessment

- Assess for medications known to inhibit the activity of microsomal oxidizing enzymes (e.g., cimetidine, isoniazid).
- Assess for medications known to intensify the CNS effect when administered with midazolam: phenothiazines, narcotics, barbiturates, MAO inhibitors, and antidepressants.
- Assess for any abnormalities in liver and kidney function.
- Assess respiratory rate, oxygen saturation, blood pressure, cardiac rate and rhythm, level of consciousness, and skin condition.

Intervention

- Slowly titrate to desired effect (i.e., initiation of slurred speech).
- Patients receiving a premedication with an opioid or other CNS depressant require less midazolam than unpremedicated patients.
- Initial titration should not exceed 2.5 mg administered over at least 2 minutes.
- Do not administer by rapid or single bolus.
- Wait an additional 2 minutes or more to evaluate effect of midazolam.
- Because the peak effect may take longer in older adult patients or those with chronic disease or decreased pulmonary reserve, an additional wait of more than 2 minutes may be indicated.
- Administer IM injection into deep muscle mass.
- Avoid intraarterial administration.
- Have suction and a positive-pressure breathing device, oxygen, and appropriate airways in the room where midazolam is to be administered.
- Have an emergency cart immediately accessible.
- The nonanesthesia provider administering midazolam should be skilled at supporting a patient's oxygenation and ventilation status.

Desired Outcome

Patient has decrease in anxiety and apprehension during procedure.
Patient has diminished recall of events during procedure.

FLUMAZENIL
(flu-MA-ze-nil)

TRADE NAME: Romazicon

CLASSIFICATION: Benzodiazepine antagonist

NOTES: Flumazenil was the first benzodiazepine antagonist available in the United States. It is indicated for complete or partial reversal of sedative benzodiazepine effects (i.e., amnestic, sedative, antianxiety, and antiseizure). Flumazenil blocks the benzodiazepine effects by competitive interaction at the benzodiazepine receptor site. It does not antagonize the effects of narcotics or other CNS agents. Flumazenil administered for a high dose of agonist (e.g., benzodiazepine overdose) will result in rapid reversal of deep CNS depression effects (i.e., loss of consciousness, respiratory depression) without disrupting the agonist effects of drowsiness and amnesia (Reves et al., 1994).

PHARMACOKINETICS: *Onset:* 30 to 60 seconds. *Peak:* 6 to 10 minutes. *Duration:* Influenced by the dose administered and the dose of the agonist. *Elimination:* Initial half-life is 7 to 17 minutes; terminal half-life is 41 to 79 minutes; hepatic metabolism; excreted in urine.

CONTRAINDICATIONS AND PRECAUTIONS: Contraindicated in patients with known hypersensitivity to flumazenil or benzodiazepines; patients undergoing long-term benzodiazepine use for a life-threatening condition (e.g., status epilepticus); and patients showing signs of serious cyclic antidepressant overdose. Use cautiously in patients with impaired hepatic or kidney function.

ADVERSE REACTIONS: *CNS:* Agitation; dizziness; emotional lability. *CV:* Cutaneous vasodilation. *GI:* Nausea and vomiting. *Other:* Shivering; pain at injection site; fatigue; blurred vision.

DOSAGE AND ADMINISTRATION
Reversal of Benzodiazepine Sedative Effects

Adult: 0.2 mg IV over 15 seconds. If the desired level of consciousness is not achieved after 45 seconds, administer another 0.2 mg. May repeat at 60-second intervals four times up to a maximum total dose of 1 mg.

Treatment of Resedation

Adult: May repeat doses administering 0.2 mg IV over 15 seconds at 20-minute intervals as needed. Administer no more than 1 mg at any one time and no more than 3 mg in any 1 hour.

Benzodiazepine Overdose

Adult: Administer 0.2 mg IV over 30 seconds; if desired level of consciousness is not achieved after 30 seconds, administer 0.3 mg over 30 seconds, waiting an additional 30 seconds to evaluate effects. Additional doses of 0.5 mg may be administered over 30 seconds at 1-minute intervals to a maximum cumulative dose of 3 mg if necessary.

NURSING CONSIDERATIONS
Assessment

- Assess patient status for long-term benzodiazepine usage.
- Assess for any abnormalities in liver and kidney function.
- Assess respiratory rate, oxygen saturation, blood pressure, cardiac rate and rhythm, level of consciousness, and skin condition.

Interventions

- Administer intravenously only; may be diluted in 5% dextrose in water, lactated Ringer's solution, and normal saline solution.
- Administer in the recommended small increments.
- To minimize patient discomfort, administer into a freely running IV line secured in a large vein.
- Monitor for signs of resedation as appropriate.

Desired Outcome
Patient has rapid return to presedation state.

OPIOIDS

General Pharmacology

The terms *opioid, opiate,* and *narcotic* are used interchangeably to describe a choice of medication administered to assist in managing pain. Proper management of pain is a critical role for the RN managing the care of a patient in a conscious sedation and analgesia state during a procedure. Several opioid analgesics are available. Those most commonly administered along with a benzodiazepine for management of conscious sedation and analgesia include morphine, fentanyl, and meperidine (Somerson, Husted, & Sicilia, 1995; Batson, 1993; Stein, 1995).

Mechanism of Action

Opioids are classified as agonists, partial agonists, mixed agonist-antagonists, and antagonists. The effects of an opioid agonist are dose dependent and occur as a result of the binding at the opioid receptor site; morphine sulfate is the prototype of a pure agonist.

Partial agonists cannot produce the full effects of a pure agonist, regardless of the dose. A mixed agonist-antagonist combines with at least one receptor from each group, producing an effect that results in management of pain with less potential for physical dependence. The antagonist (i.e., naloxone) produces no effects but displaces other agonists at the receptor sites and directly reverses respiratory depression, analgesia, drowsiness, and other effects of the agonists and agonist-antagonists.

The actions of opioids are determined by the target-cell receptors, which are known as opioid receptor sites. These sites are primarily located in the CNS. The opioid receptor sites are labeled by the prototype agonist that produces its distinct properties (e.g., mu for morphine, kappa for ketocyclazocine, and sigma for SKF10 047-*N*-allylnormetazocine) (Bovill, 1988). Bailey and Stanley (1994, p. 297) report the major actions of opioid receptors, which include the following: mu receptors produce analgesia, respiratory depression, physical dependence, euphoria and bradycardia; kappa receptors produce weak analgesia, respiratory depression, and sedation; sigma receptors produce dysphoria/delirium mydriasis, hallucinations, tachycardia, and hypertension; and delta receptors produce weak analgesia and respiratory depression.

Pharmacokinetics

The pure agonists opioids are dose related and may produce respiratory depression. Respiratory depression generally occurs within 5 to 10 minutes following IV injection, with duration dependent on the medication's half-life. The patient with

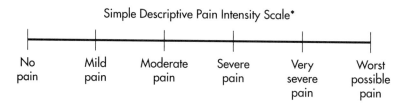

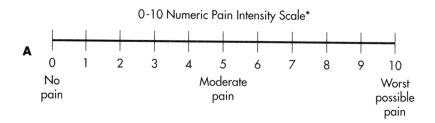

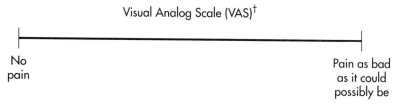

*If used as a graphic rating scale, a 10-cm baseline is recommended.
†A 10-cm baseline is recommended for VAS scales.

FIGURE 3-2 | **A,** Pain intensity scales. (From AHCPR–Acute Pain Management Guideline Panel. [February, 1992]. *Acute pain management: Operative or medical procedures and trauma. Clinical practice guideline.* [AHCPR Pub. No. 92-0032]. Rockville, MD: Agency for Health Care Policy and Research, Public Health Service, U.S. Department of Health and Human Services.)

depressed respirations from opioid administration may respond to command (i.e., take a deep breath) or stimulation. If respirations are not adequate to increase and maintain adequate ventilation and oxygenation, an opioid-antagonist may be administered to reverse the respiratory depression and analgesia. Most opioids are broken down by hepatic metabolism into greatly reduced opioid metabolites.

Clinical Use

Opioids may be administered as a premedication or along with another medication, generally a benzodiazepine, during the procedure. To provide optimal management of pain during the procedure, a pain history should be obtained. The pain history should include the following information: how the patient reacts to pain;

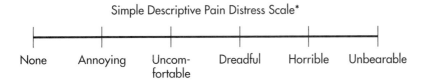

Simple Descriptive Pain Distress Scale*

None   Annoying   Uncom-   Dreadful   Horrible   Unbearable
                    fortable

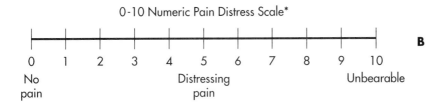

0-10 Numeric Pain Distress Scale*

0   1   2   3   4   5   6   7   8   9   10   **B**
No   Distressing   Unbearable
pain   pain

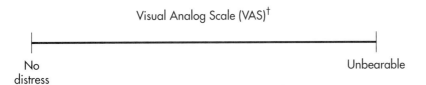

Visual Analog Scale (VAS)†

No   Unbearable
distress

*If used as a graphic rating scale, a 10-cm baseline is recommended.
†A 10-cm baseline is recommended for VAS scales.

FIGURE 3-2 | B, Pain distress scales. (From AHCPR–Acute Pain Management Guideline Panel. [February, 1992]. *Acute pain management: Operative or medical procedures and trauma. Clinical practice guideline.* [AHCPR Pub. No. 92-0032]. Rockville, MD: Agency for Health Care Policy and Research, Public Health Service, U.S. Department of Health and Human Services.)

previous methods that were found to be effective in managing pain; the patient's attitude toward the use of opioids, anxiolytics, and other medications; identification of substance abuse; the patient's usual response to pain; how the patient communicates pain, and the extent of pain management the patient expects during the procedure (AHCPR). There are a variety of methods to assess pain. The most commonly used during a short-term therapeutic, diagnostic, or surgical procedure are the pain intensity scales (Figure 3-2).

Opioids are effective in elevating the pain threshold. Most often an opioid and a benzodiazapine are administered along with local or regional anesthesia. The local anesthesia agent blocks transmission of the pain impulse. However, there are procedures for which local anesthesia is not appropriate, and the administration of an opioid will allow pain to be felt as distant or dislocated (Somerson, Husted, & Sicilia, 1995). The patient should be aware that the sensations of tugging, pressure, and pulling are common.

BUTORPHANOL TARTRATE
(byou-TOR-fah-nohl)

TRADE NAME: Stadol

CLASSIFICATION: Narcotic agonist-antagonist, opioid partial agonist

NOTES: Butorphanol has been available in the United States since 1979. It has both agonist and antagonist properties. Butorphanol is not a controlled substance and is less likely to be abused and cause dependency than narcotics. The administration of 2 mg IV is comparable to 10 mg IV of morphine. Vogelsang and Hayes (1991) report that butorphanol tartrate has strong kappa receptor activation (i.e., marked sedation) and sigma receptor activation (i.e., stimulation of respiratory drive). It has mu receptor antagonism and is not recommended for the patient taking narcotic agents. Because butorphanol is an agonist/antagonist medication, the risk of respiratory depression is greatly reduced when compared to the effects of a narcotic agonist such as meperidine, fentanyl, or morphine.

PHARMACOKINETICS: *Onset:* 2 to 3 minutes IV; 10 to 30 minutes IM. *Peak:* 30 minutes IV; 30 to 60 minutes IM. *Duration:* 2 to 4 hours. *Metabolism:* Occurs in the liver. *Elimination:* Half-life is 2.15 to 3.5 hours; excreted in urine and bile.

CONTRAINDICATIONS AND PRECAUTIONS: Contraindicated in patients with known hypersensitivity to butorphanol tartrate. Administer with caution to any patient with supraventricular dysrhythmias, renal or hepatic dysfunction, pulmonary disease (e.g., asthma, chronic obstructive pulmonary disease [COPD]), convulsive disorders, or physical addiction to narcotics. The drug may cause biliary spasm and seizures in patients with convulsive disorders. Administer cautiously in hypertensive patients because hypertension may result.

ADVERSE REACTIONS: *CNS:* Sedation; headache; vertigo; lethargy; dizziness; confusion; lightheadedness. *CV:* Palpitations; hypotension; hypertension. *GI:* Nausea; vomiting; dry mouth. *Skin:* Rash; flushing; clamminess and excessive sweating. *Other:* Respiratory depression.

DOSAGE AND ADMINISTRATION
Premedication
Adult: 2 mg IM 60 to 90 minutes before procedure.

Intravenous Conscious Sedation
Adult: 0.5 to 2 mg IV every 3 to 4 hours.

NURSING CONSIDERATIONS

Assessment

- Assess patient's medication history for possible interactions with other CNS depressant medications that the patient may be taking.
- Assess for history of drug dependence, which can precipitate withdrawal symptoms.
- Assess and choose with patient an appropriate pain intensity scale.
- Assess for kidney and liver dysfunction.
- Assess baseline monitoring data: respiratory rate, oxygen saturation, blood pressure, cardiac rate and rhythm, level of consciousness, and skin condition.

Intervention

- If administering with another CNS depressant, decrease dose by 30%.

Desired Outcome

- Patient has safe administration of medication.
- Patient demonstrates adequate pain management.

MEPERIDINE HYDROCHLORIDE

(me-PER-i-deen)

TRADE NAME: Demerol

CLASSIFICATION: Narcotic analgesic, opioid

NOTES: Meperidine causes histamine release at a greater frequency than do other opioids. It has atropine-like effects, and the patient may experience tachycardia following IV administration.

PHARMACOKINETICS: *Onset:* 1 to 5 minutes IV; 15 minutes PO; 10 minutes IM. *Peak:* 10 to 20 minutes IV; 1 hour PO; 1 hour IM. *Duration:* 1 to 2 hours. *Elimination:* Half-life is 2 to 6 hours; metabolized by hydrolysis in liver; excreted in urine.

CONTRAINDICATIONS AND PRECAUTIONS: Contraindicated in patients with known hypersensitivity to meperidine or other phenylpiperidine opioids. Administer with caution to any patient with supraventricular dysrhythmias, head injury, renal or hepatic dysfunction, pulmonary disease, convulsive disorder or glaucoma and to older adult or debilitated patients. May interact with MAO inhibitors and result in hypertension, excitation, tachycardia, seizure, and hyperpyrexia (Vissering, 1993).

ADVERSE REACTIONS: *CNS:* Drowsiness; dizziness; confusion; headache; sedation; euphoria; convulsions at high doses. *CV:* Tachycardia; asystole; bradycardia; palpitations; hypotension; syncope. *GI:* Nausea; vomiting; anorexia; constipation; cramps. *Skin:* Rash; urticaria; bruising; flushing; diaphoresis; pruritus. *EENT:* Tinnitus; blurred vision; miosis; diplopia. *Resp:* Respiratory depression.

DOSAGE AND ADMINISTRATION
Premedication
Adult: 50 to 100 mg IM or SC 30 to 90 minutes before procedure. *Pediatric:* 1 to 3 mg/kg IM or SC 30 to 90 minutes before procedure.

Intravenous Conscious Sedation
Adult: 15 to 35 mg IV before procedure. *Pediatric:* 1 to 3 mg/kg IV.

NURSING CONSIDERATIONS
Assessment
- Assess patient's medication history for current use of MAO inhibitors (i.e., isocarboxazid, pargyline, phenelzine, and tranylcypromine).
- Assess for history of drug dependence.
- Assess and choose with patient an appropriate pain intensity scale.
- Assess for kidney and liver dysfunction.
- Assess baseline monitoring data: respiratory rate, oxygen saturation, blood pressure, cardiac rate and rhythm, level of consciousness, and skin condition.

Intervention
- Administer slowly over 30 seconds or longer into an infusing IV line. Injectable meperidine is compatible with normal saline, dextrose 5%, lactated Ringer's solution, and sodium lactate solution.
- May be administered to some patients with known sensitivity to morphine.
- For drug overdose administer narcotic antagonist (naloxone).
- Administer 25% to 50% less if administered with another CNS depressant.
- For nausea and vomiting administer an antiemetic (e.g., droperidol, compazine).

Desired Outcome
- Patient has safe administration of medication.
- Patient demonstrates adequate pain management.

FENTANYL CITRATE
(FEN-tah-nil)

TRADE NAME: Sublimaze

CLASSIFICATION: Opioid

NOTES: Fentanyl is a popular opioid used as a supplement in balanced anesthesia. It is frequently administered as an agent for sedation and analgesia because of its short-acting effects, which are similar to those of morphine and meperidine. Fentanyl is usually administered following a benzodiazepine and is rapidly dissolved in highly perfused tissue and stored in fat and muscle tissue (Willens, 1994). When fentanyl is released from fat and muscle tissue back into circulation, delayed-onset respiratory depression may result. A dose of 100 μg is equivalent in analgesic activity to 10 mg of morphine or 75 mg of meperidine.

PHARMACOKINETICS: *Onset:* 1 to 3 minutes IV; 7 to 8 minutes IM. *Peak:* 5 to 15 minutes IV. *Metabolism:* Occurs in liver. *Duration:* 30 to 60 min following single IV dose less than 100 μg. *Elimination:* Half-life is 4 hours; excreted in urine.

CONTRAINDICATIONS AND PRECAUTIONS: Contraindicated in patients with known hypersensitivity to fentanyl. Administer with caution to any patient with supraventricular dysrhythmias or bradycardia, head injury, renal or hepatic dysfunction, pulmonary disease (e.g., asthma, COPD), convulsive disorders, or physical addiction to this medication. It is not recommended for patients taking MAO inhibitors 14 days before administration. Use with other CNS depressant medications should include decreased administration of fentanyl by one quarter to one third.

ADVERSE REACTIONS: *CNS:* Sedation; dizziness; delirium; seizures; euphoria. *GI:* Nausea; vomiting. *EENT:* Blurred vision; miosis. *CV:* Bradycardia; tachycardia; palpitations; arrest; hypertension; hypotension. *Resp:* Respiratory depression; arrest; laryngospasm. *Other:* Apnea; skeletal muscle rigidity.

DOSAGE AND ADMINISTRATION
Premedication
Adult: 0.05 to 0.1 mg IM 30 to 60 minutes before procedure.

Intravenous Conscious Sedation
Adult: 0.05 to 2 μg/kg IV titrated to patient response.

NURSING CONSIDERATIONS
Assessment
- Assess patient's medication history for current use of MAO inhibitors (i.e., isocarboxazid, pargyline, phenelzine, and tranylcypromine).
- Assess for history of drug dependence.
- Assess and choose with patient an appropriate pain intensity scale.
- Assess to determine if patient is taking calcium channel blockers, beta blockers, benzodiazepines, or tranquilizers, which could cause severe hypotension.
- Assess for kidney or liver dysfunction.
- Assess baseline monitoring data: respiratory rate, oxygen saturation, blood pressure, cardiac rate and rhythm, level of consciousness, and skin condition.

Intervention

- Patient may receive an anticholinergic (e.g., atropine) preprocedure to minimize the effect of bradycardia.
- Administer in slow incremental doses of 25 to 50 µg at 1 to 2 minute intervals, titrated to patient response.
- Apnea and muscle rigidity could pose a problem; be prepared to treat with assisted ventilation and naloxone.
- If administering with another CNS depressant, decrease dose by 30%.

Desired Outcome

- Patient has safe administration of medication.
- Patient demonstrates adequate pain management.

MORPHINE SULFATE
(MOR-feen)

TRADE NAMES: Astromorph PF, Duramorph PF, MS Contin, Roxanol

CLASSIFICATION: Narcotic analgesic, opioid

NOTES: Morphine is a commonly administered opioid. Morphine may be titrated to the desired patient effect and is reversible with naloxone hydrochloride. It has a high affinity for mu and kapa receptors and produces excellent alterations in pain perception and emotional response.

PHARMACOKINETICS: *Onset:* 1 to 3 minutes IV. *Peak:* 10 to 20 minutes IV. *Metabolism:* Occurs in liver. *Duration:* 1 to 2 hours. *Elimination:* Half-life is 3 to 7 hours; excreted in urine and bile.

CONTRAINDICATIONS AND PRECAUTIONS: Contraindicated in patients with known hypersensitivity to morphine or phenanthrene opioids (i.e., codeine, hydrocodone, hydromorphone, oxycodone, oxymorphone). Administer with caution to any patient with supraventricular dysrhythmias, head injury or increased intercranial pressure and any pregnant patient. Administer cautiously in patients with renal or hepatic dysfunction, pulmonary disease (e.g., asthma, COPD), convulsive disorders, or physical addiction to this medication. Concomitant use with other CNS-depressant medications potentiates the effects; decrease normal dose by one quarter to one third.

ADVERSE REACTIONS: *CNS:* Sedation; dizziness; delirium; seizures; euphoria. *GI:* Nausea; vomiting; constipation. *GU:* Urinary retention. *EENT:* Blurred vision; miosis. *CV:* Bradycardia; tachycardia; palpitations; asystole; hypertension; hypotension. *Resp:* Respiratory depression. *Other:* Rash, urticaria, flushing; diaphoresis.

DOSAGE AND ADMINISTRATION

Intravenous Conscious Sedation

Adult: 2.5 to 10 mg IV. *Pediatric:* 0.05 to 0.1 mg/kg IV.

NURSING CONSIDERATIONS

Assessment

- Assess patient's medication history for possible interactions with other CNS-depressant medications that the patient may be taking.
- Assess for history of drug dependence.
- Assess and choose with patient an appropriate pain intensity scale.
- Assess for kidney and liver dysfunction.
- Assess baseline monitoring data: respiratory rate, oxygen saturation, blood pressure, cardiac rate and rhythm, level of consciousness, and skin condition.

Intervention

- Administer slowly over 4 to 5 minutes; may be diluted with water for injection.
- If administering with another CNS depressant, decrease dose by 30%.

Desired Outcome

- Patient has safe administration of medication.
- Patient demonstrates adequate pain management.

NALBUPHINE HYDROCHLORIDE

(NAL-byoo-feen)

TRADE NAME: Nubain

CLASSIFICATION: Narcotic agonist-antagonist, opioid partial agonist

NOTES: This drug is a potent analgesic with narcotic agonists and antagonist actins. Its analgesic potency is equivalent to that of morphine.

PHARMACOKINETICS: *Onset:* 2 to 3 minutes IV. *Peak:* 30 to 60 minutes IV. *Metabolism:* Occurs in liver. *Duration:* 3 to 6 hours. *Elimination:* Half-life is 3 to 7 hours; excreted in urine and bile.

CONTRAINDICATIONS AND PRECAUTIONS: Contraindicated in patients with known hypersensitivity to nalbuphine hydrochloride or other phenanthrene opioids (i.e., codeine, hydrocodone, hydromorphone, oxycodone, oxymorphone). Administer with caution to any patient with supraventricular dysrhythmias, head injury, or increased intracranial pressure. Administer cautiously in patients with renal or hepatic dysfunction, pulmonary disease (e.g., asthma, COPD), or physical addiction to this medication. Other CNS depressants may potentiate the effects of the medication.

DOSAGE AND ADMINISTRATION
Intravenous Conscious Sedation
Adult: 10 to 20 mg IV every 3 to 6 hours.

NURSING CONSIDERATIONS
Assessment
- Assess patient's medication history for possible interactions with other CNS-depressant medications that the patient may be taking.
- Assess for allergies to sulfites; drug contains sodium metabisulfite as a preservative and should not be administered to patients with such allergy.
- Assess for history of drug dependence.
- Assess and choose with patient an appropriate pain intensity scale.
- Assess for kidney and liver dysfunction.
- Assess baseline monitoring data: respiratory rate, oxygen saturation, blood pressure, cardiac rate and rhythm, level of consciousness, and skin condition.

Intervention
- Administer slowly over 3 to 5 minutes. Usual recommended dose for 70 kg is 10 mg.
- If administering with another CNS depressant, decrease dose by 30%.

Desired Outcome
- Patient has safe administration of medication.
- Patient demonstrates adequate pain management.

NALOXONE HYDROCHLORIDE
(nal-OX-ohn)

TRADE NAME: Narcan

CLASSIFICATION: Narcotic antagonist

NOTES: Introduced in the 1960s for rapid reversal of opioid-induced respiratory depression. It is active at mu, delta, kappa, and sigma receptors. For most patients naloxone antagonizes the opioid effects of respiratory depression, apnea, and sedation. It has a short duration of action, which is usually shorter than that of most opioids.

PHARMACOKINETICS: *Onset:* 1 to 2 minutes IV; 2 to 5 minutes IM or SC. *Peak:* 5 to 15 minutes IV. *Metabolism:* Occurs in liver by conjugation. *Duration:* 45 minutes. *elimination:* Half-life is 30 to 90 minutes; excreted in urine.

CONTRAINDICATIONS AND PRECAUTIONS: Contraindicated in patients with known hypersensitivity to naloxone. If this drug is administered to a patient with opioid drug dependence, severe withdrawal syndrome may result. Administer with caution to patients with supraventricular dysrhythmias, head injuries, or convulsive disorders.

DOSAGE AND ADMINISTRATION: *Adult:* Narcotic overdose: 0.4 to 2 mg IV/SC/IM every 2 to 3 minutes as needed. Reversal of postoperative narcotic depression: 0.1 to 0.2 mg IV/SC/IM every 2 to 3 minutes as needed.

NURSING CONSIDERATIONS

Assessment

- Obtain a true history from patient to determine narcotic addiction.
- Continued assessment is necessary following administration because of the shorter duration of action than that of the opioid.
- Determine narcotic half-life and compare to half-life of naloxone.

Intervention

- Monitor respiratory and cardiovascular function.
- Document reason for administration.

Desired Outcome

- Patient has reversal of respiratory depression related to narcotic overdose.

OTHER MEDICATIONS

Although the following medications do not fall into the classification of a benzodiazepine or opioid, they are frequently administered as part of the pharmacology regimen for conscious sedation and analgesia.

PROPOFOL

(PRO-po-fol)

TRADE NAME: Diprivan

CLASSIFICATION: General anesthetic

NOTES: Propofol has been available since November 1989. It is an IV anesthetic administered for induction and maintenance of anesthesia, for sedation of the mechanically ventilated ICU patient, and as supplementation to local anesthesia.

Propofol has a rapid onset of action, short duration, and hypnotic and antiemetic effects. It is an emulsion-based product mixed with soybean oil, glycerol, and egg phosphatide. If diluted, it is compatible with 5% dextrose in water.

PHARMACOKINETICS: *Onset:* 30 to 45 seconds. *Peak:* 92 seconds. *Duration:* 1.8 to 8.3 minutes for distribution phase; 34 to 64 minutes for second distribution; and 3 to 8 hours for terminal elimination. *Elimination:* Extrahepatic metabolism and/or extrarenal elimination; metabolized in the liver and excreted by the kidneys; metabolites are not active.

CONTRAINDICATIONS AND PRECAUTIONS: Known hypersensitivity to propofol. Should be administered only by persons trained in the techniques of general anesthesia, except in the ICU, where the patient is intubated and mechanically ventilated.

ADVERSE REACTIONS: *CNS:* Movement; headache; dizziness; twitching; clonic/myoclonic movement. *CV:* Hypotension; hypertension; bradycardia. *GI:* Nausea; vomiting; cramping. *Resp:* Apnea; cough; hiccup. *Skin:* Flushing. *Other:* Injection site pain.

DOSAGE AND ADMINISTRATION
Continuous Infusion for Sedation in ICU

Adult (IV): Doucet, Rabbett, and Barsanti (1995) recommend titration to individual response. *Initial dose:* Administer 5 µg/kg/min (0.3 mg/kg/hr) IV over 5 or more minutes. *Additional increments:* Administer in increments of 5 to 10 µg/kg/min (0.3-0.6 mg/kg/hr) IV over 5 to 10 minutes until desired level of sedation is achieved. *Maintenance:* Infusion of 5 to 50 µg/kg/min (0.3-3 mg/kg/hr) IV.

NURSING CONSIDERATIONS
Assessment

- Assess for appropriate pain management; propofol has no analgesic properties.
- Assess that appropriate emergency resuscitative equipment is immediately available.

Intervention

- Dilute with 5% dextrose injection. May be administered into infusing IV line with 5% dextrose injection, lactated Ringer's injection, lactated Ringer's and 5% dextrose injection, 5% dextrose and 0.45% sodium chloride injection, and 5% dextrose and 0.2% sodium chloride injection.
- Discard any unused portion after 6 hours (if diluted) or 12 hours (if used directly from vial).
- Administer into large veins (e.g., forearm, antecubital fossa).
- Use strict aseptic technique; propofol contains no preservatives or antimicrobial agents.

Desired Outcome
- ICU patient has safe administration of medication.
- ICU patient demonstrates adequate level of sedation.

KETAMINE
(KEET-a-meen)

TRADE NAME: Ketalar

CLASSIFICATION: General anesthetic

NOTES: Ketamine administration results in dissociative anesthesia. The patient is dissociated from the environment and may appear to be in a dreamlike cataleptic state and can follow simple commands. There is controversy regarding the administration of this agent by a nonanesthesia provider for conscious sedation and analgesia during short-term therapeutic, diagnostic, or surgical procedures. Recovery time may be prolonged because of emergence reactions from ketamine (e.g., dreams, hallucinations, and delirium).

PHARMACOKINETICS: *Onset:* 30 seconds IV; 3 to 4 minutes IM. *Peak:* 1 minute IV; 5 minutes IM. *Duration:* 5 to 10 minutes IV; 12 to 25 minutes IM. *Metabolism:* Metabolized by liver enzymes. *Elimination:* Half-life is 2 to 3 hours; excreted in urine.

CONTRAINDICATIONS AND PRECAUTIONS: Do not administer if known hypersensitivity to ketamine is present. Contraindicated for patients diagnosed with schizophrenia or other acute psychiatric disorders and hypertension.

ADVERSE REACTIONS: *CNS:* Confusion; excitement; irrational behavior; hallucinations; excitement; dreamlike state. *CV:* Hypertension; hypotension; tachycardia. *EENT:* Excessive salivation; diplopia; laryngospasm. *GI:* Nausea; vomiting. *Skin:* Rash.

DOSAGE AND ADMINISTRATION: *Adult: IV:* 1 to 4.5 mg/kg over 1 minute; *IM:* 6.5 to 13 mg/kg. *Pediatric:* 1 to 3 mg/kg.

NURSING CONSIDERATIONS
Assessment
- Assess for kidney and liver dysfunction.
- Assess baseline monitoring data: respiratory rate, oxygen saturation, blood pressure, cardiac rate and rhythm, level of consciousness, and skin condition.
- Assess for patent infusing IV line.

Intervention
- Dilute with equal amount of sterile water, normal saline, or 5% dextrose in water.
- Because of rapid onset of action and short clinical effect, administration may be done after draping is complete.

- Have emergency cart with equipment and medications immediately available.
- Frequently monitor patient's vital signs (e.g., every 5 to 15 minutes).
- During recovery keep verbal communication and tactile stimulation to a minimum to minimize emergence reactions (i.e., dreams, visual imagery, hallucinations, and delirium).
- Have diazepam immediately available; may be administered to decrease incidence of emergence reactions.

Desired Outcome

- Patient has safe administration of medication.

CONCLUSION

The RN should be knowledgeable about the medications, recommended dosages, and potential adverse effects of the medications that he or she may administer to patients. Each institution should have clearly defined techniques in which the nonanesthesia provider administers the medications under the direction of a physician. To safely administer these and other medications to achieve a state of conscious sedation and analgesia, the nonanesthesia provider must obtain relevant knowledge and training to allow for safe and proper administration.

REFERENCES

Bailey, P. L., & Stanley, T. H. (1994). Intravenous opioid anesthetics. In R. D. Miller (Ed.), *Anesthesia* (4th ed., Vol 1). New York: Churchill Livingstone.

Batson, V. D. (1993). Conscious sedation: Implications for perioperative nursing practice. *Seminars in Perioperative Nursing, 2*(1), 45-57.

Bovill, J. G. (1988). The opioids in intravenous anaesthesia. In J. W. Dundee & G. M. Wyant. (Eds.), *Intravenous Anesthesia* (pp. 206-247). New York: Churchill Livingstone.

Doucet, M. A., Rabbett, P., & Barsanti, F. (1995). Administering I. V. sedatives. *Nursing 95, 25*(4), 32RR-32SS.

Reves, J. G., Glass, P. S., & Lubarsky, D. A. (1994). In R. D. Miller (Ed.), *Anesthesia* (Vol. 1, pp. 248-259). New York: Churchill Livingstone.

Shannon, M. T., Wilson, B. A., & Stang, C. (1995). *Drugs and nursing implications* (8th ed.). Norwalk, CT: Appleton & Lange.

Somerson, S. J., Husted, C. W., & Sicilia, M. R. (1995). Insights into conscious sedation. *American Journal of Nursing, 95*(6), 26-32.

Stein R. (1995). The perioperative nurse's role in anesthesia management. *AORN Journal, 62*(5), 794-804.

Sternbach, L. H. (1978). The benzodiazepine story. *Progress in Drug Research, 22,* 229-266.

Vogelsang, J., & Hayes, S. R. (1991). Butorphanol tartrate (stadol): A review. *Journal of Post Anesthesia Nursing, 6*(2), 129-135.

Willens, J. S. (1994). Giving fentanyl for pain outside the OR. *American Journal of Nursing,* February, pp. 24-28.

BIBLIOGRAPHY

Bell, J., Sartain, J., Wilkinson, G., & Sherry, K. (1994). Propofol and fentanyl anesthesia for patients with low cardiac output state undergoing cardiac surgery: comparison with high-dose fentanyl anaesthesia. *British Journal of Anaesthesia, 73*, 162-166.

Bennett et al. (1995). Postoperative infections traced to contamination of an intravenous anesthetic, propofol. *The New England Journal of Medicine, 333*(3), 184-185.

Claussen, D. W. (1994). Endoscopy nursing education competency: Romazicon administration for IV conscious sedation reversal. *Gastroenterology Nursing, 17*(3), 121-123.

Claussen, D. W. (1994). Versed administration for IV conscious sedation. *Gastroenterology Nursing, 17*(2), 80-84.

Carrasco, G., Molina, R., Costa, J., Soler, J., Cabré, L. (1993). Propofol vs midazolam in short-, medium-, and long-term sedation of critically ill patients. *Chest, 103*(3), 557-564.

Dundee, J. W., & Wyant, G. M. (1988). The benzodiazepines. In J. W. Dundee & G. M. Wyant (Eds.), *Intravenous Anesthesia* (pp. 184-205). New York: Churchill Livingstone.

Glover, D. G., & Lopez, J. R. (1995). Clinical drug evaluation: Flumazenil. *Federal Practitioner, 12*, 34-49.

Hayes, S. R., & Vogelsang, J. (1991). Opiate receptors and analgesia: An update. *Journal of Post Anesthesia Nursing, 6*(2), 125-128.

Higgins, T.L., Yared, J., Estafanous, F.G., Coyle, J.P., Ko, H.K., Goodale, D.B. (1994). Propofol versus midazolam for intensive care unit sedation after coronary artery bypass grafting. *Critical Care Medicine, 22*(9), 1415-1423.

Holloran, T., & Pohlman, A. S. (1995). Managing sedation in the critically ill patient. *Critical Care Nurse, 15*(4 Suppl), 1-14; quiz 15-6.

Idemoto, B. K. (1995). Propofol: A new treatment in intensive care unit sedation. *AACN Clinical Issues, 6*(2), 333-343.

Jensen, D. (1995). Applying a sedation algorithm to ICU patients in pain. *Dimensions Critical Care Nursing, 14*(2), 67-68.

Malamed, S. F. (1995). *Sedation: A guide to patient management* (3rd ed.). St. Louis: Mosby.

Maree, S. M. (1992). Benzodiazepines and their reversal. *Current Reviews for Nurse Anesthetists, 15*(7), 53-60.

Markee, S. M. (1992). Benzodiazepines and their reversal. *Current Reviews for Nurse Anesthetists* 15(7), 53-60.

Ringler, J. D. (1995). The use of diazepam and ketamine for IV conscious sedation in outpatient surgery settings. *AORN Journal, 62*(4), 638-645.

Spratto, G. R., & Woods, A. L. (1996). *PDR nurse's handbook.* Montvale, NJ: Medical Economics.

Vissering, T.R. (1993). Narcotics and implications for the post anesthesia care unit. *Nursing Clinics of North America, 28*(3), 573-579.

Westcott, D. The sedation of patients in intensive care units: A nursing review. *Intensive Critical Care Nursing, 11*(1), 26-31.

Whitman, M. (1995). The push is on delivering medications safely by IV bolus. *Nursing 95, 25*(8), 52-54.

Management of Complications

Although intravenous (IV) conscious sedation and analgesia permits rapid recovery from short-term therapeutic, diagnostic, and surgical procedures and poses less danger to the patient than does general anesthesia, it has its hazards. Complications can arise from the use of any level of sedation and analgesia, and the patient's outcome depends on the ability of health care personnel to identify and treat these complications. Because IV conscious sedation and analgesia is usually used during "minor" surgical and medical procedures, many caregivers may be unprepared for and may underestimate the complications that may occur. The lack of awareness may result in delayed response and negative patient outcome. Many clinicians erroneously assume that patients may be too "sick" for general anesthesia but not for IV conscious sedation and analgesia (Fallacaro, 1993). This sets the stage for unanticipated complications that are not identified or treated in a proactive manner.

Because IV conscious sedation and analgesia is being used outside the traditional surgical suite in less controlled settings, such as ambulatory care, surgical and endoscopy suites, cardiac catheterization laboratories, emergency and radiology departments, and even physician offices, greater vigilance in patient monitoring is required. Most of the procedures for which IV conscious sedation and analgesia is being used do not require the presence of an anesthesiologist. Such procedures include wound dressing changes, bronchoscopy, endoscopy, cardioversion, cardiac catheterization, treatment of simple fractures, and dental procedures (Somerson, Husted, & Sicilia, 1995). Therefore registered nurses (RNs) who do not exclusively specialize in conscious sedation and anesthesia must understand the care required. Because the procedures for which conscious sedation and analgesia is being administered can be uncomfortable, analgesics (opioids) and sedatives (benzodiazepines) are administered simultaneously. The opioids commonly used are morphine, fentanyl, and meperidine. At standard doses for IV administration, opioids induce analgesia without disturbing protective reflexes or ventilation. The most common sedatives used in IV conscious sedation and analgesia are the benzodiazepines (midazolam and diazepam). These agents reduce anxiety and induce short-term amnesia. Also at standard doses they do not interfere with protective reflexes and breathing. However, when sedatives and analgesics are administered simultaneously, the potential for complications increases (Reves, Glass, & Lubarsky, 1995).

To be able to safely care for patients undergoing IV conscious sedation and analgesia, RNs must understand the effects of all the drugs used (i.e., sedatives, analgesics, and reversal agents). In addition, the RN must understand the desired goals of IV conscious sedation and analgesia, the consequences of deeper levels of sedation, and the rapid assessment and treatment of the most common complications. The patient who has received IV conscious sedation and analgesia should experience a decreased level of consciousness but should retain the ability to independently and continuously maintain a patent airway and respond appropriately to verbal commands and/or physical stimulation (American Nurses Association, 1991). During IV conscious sedation and analgesia, vital signs remain stable. As the patient progresses toward general anesthesia, cardiac, respiratory, and reflex functions become altered to the extent of requiring external support. At this juncture the patient's care becomes much more complex (beyond the scope of an RN) and necessitates the expertise of an anesthesiologist (Proudfoot, 1995).

IV CONSCIOUS SEDATION AND ANALGESIA: NOT A BENIGN TREATMENT

IV conscious sedation and analgesia is not a treatment without consequence. In 1982 the first report on morbidity and mortality data in dental patients receiving IV conscious sedation stated that airway obstruction, unrelieved hypoxemia, and cardiac events were among the leading causes of death (Coplans & Curson, 1982). In 1986 the U.S. Food and Drug Administration received reports of 66 deaths that occurred during IV conscious sedation and analgesia outside the surgical suite. Cardiopulmonary depression was cited as the most common cause of death (Fallacaro, 1993). In 1990 more than 80 deaths were attributed to the benzodiazepines and opioids used during IV conscious sedation and analgesia (Bailey et al., 1990). A 1991 study focused on patients who underwent dental and oral maxillofacial procedures involving IV conscious sedation and analgesia. The study established that most adverse events in this patient population were related to preexisting comorbidities that could have been avoided with more intensive monitoring (Jastak & Peskin, 1991). Unfortunately, even after the publication of these results, many physicians will have not changed their practice to include preventive measures. A 1991 survey of 32 dental practices revealed that approximately half of those administering IV conscious sedation did not have reversal agents available for management of overdose (Luyk & Ferguson, 1993).

The lack of attention on the prevention of complications has prompted medical and nursing organizations to publish guidelines and recommendations for the care of patients undergoing IV conscious sedation and analgesia. (See Appendixes A through F.) In an attempt to minimize complications related to the use of IV conscious sedation and analgesia, a position statement published by the American

Nurses Association and endorsed by 23 specialty nursing organizations. This position statement says that the RN caring for the patient should be able to "assess total patient care requirements during IV conscious sedation and recovery." To meet these needs, the RN must be able to "anticipate and recognize potential complications of IV conscious sedation in relation to the type of medication being administered." Finally, the RN must "possess the knowledge and skills to assess, diagnose, and intervene in the event of complications or undesired outcomes" (American Nurses Association, 1991). The same competencies are required by the Joint Commission on Accreditation of Healthcare Organizations (JCAHO, 1996). Box 4-1 focuses on the knowledge necessary to prevent or treat complications. It can be used as a quick reference to assess skills of RNs caring for patients undergoing IV conscious sedation and analgesia.

BOX 4-1 *Registered Nurse Competencies for IV Conscious Sedation and Analgesia*

I. Pharmacology of medications commonly administered
  A. Benzodiazepines
  B. Opioids
  C. Reversal agents
II. Management of potential complications
  A. Neurologic
    1. Undersedation
    2. Oversedation
  B. Cardiovascular
    1. Dysrhythmia—recognition and management
      a. Antidysrhythmics
      b. Defibrillation
      c. Cardiopulmonary resuscitation
    2. Hemodynamic instability—recognition and management
      a. Fluid resuscitation
      b. Inotropes
    3. Myocardial ischemia/infarction—recognition and management
  C. Respiratory
    1. Airway compromise—recognition and management
      a. Head tilt–chin lift maneuver
      b. Intubation
    2. Resuscitative oxygenation/ventilation
      a. Oxygen delivery devices
      b. Bag-and-mask ventilation

PREVENTION

The key to prevention of overdose and other potential complications associated with IV conscious sedation and analgesia is vigilant monitoring. In addition to the level of consciousness, principal patient physiologic variables such as respiratory rate and rhythm, oxygen saturation, cardiac rate and rhythm, and blood pressure should be assessed frequently. Early detection of a variation from the norm may avert the occurrence of an adverse effect. See Table 4-1 for the normal values of vital signs commonly noted during monitoring with IV conscious sedation and analgesia (Stevens & White, 1995).

TABLE 4-1 *Age-Specific Vital Signs*

VITAL SIGN	AGE	BREATHS/MIN	
Respiratory rate	Infants (6 mo)	30-60	
	Toddlers (2 yr)	24-40	
	Preschoolers (5 yr)	22-34	
	School-aged children (7 yr)	18-30	
	Adolescents (15 yr)	12-16	
	Adults (>18 yr)	10-20	
	AGE	PERCENTAGE	
Oxygen saturation	All ages	95-100	
	AGE	BEATS/MIN	
Heart rate	Infants	120-160	
	Toddlers	90-140	
	Preschoolers	80-110	
	School-aged children	75-100	
	Adolescents	60-90	
	Adults	60-100	
	Athletes	50-100	
	AGE	SYSTOLIC	DIASTOLIC
Blood pressure	Infants	87-105	53-66
	Toddlers	95-105	53-66
	School-aged children	97-112	57-71
	Adolescents	112-128	66-80
	Adults	100-140	60-80

Modified from Daily, E., Schroeder, J. (1994). *Techniques in bedside hemodynamic monitoring.* St. Louis: Mosby.

HIGH-RISK PATIENTS

Through identification of high-risk patients, certain complications can be anticipated. Before the procedure the RN must assess the patient's medical history to identify comorbidities that could predispose the patient to certain adverse events. The medical history regarding the patient's response to sedation and analgesia will also assist the nurse in averting preventable complications.

Since older adults have a larger proportion of fat to total body weight, highly lipophilic sedatives such as benzodiazepines have prolonged elimination half-lives in such patients (Esch, 1995). Therefore reducing the dose of benzodiazepine in patients older than age 60 by 50% should be considered (Claussen, 1994). Because of the potential for prolonged sedation, the duration of postprocedure monitoring should also be lengthened. On the other end of the age spectrum, children with certain cardiopulmonary disorders also require special attention since they may undergo desaturation rapidly after sedation (Cote, 1995).

Benzodiazepines are metabolized by the liver. Any cause of liver dysfunction, such as structural liver disease, congestive heart failure, or shock, can result in the slower elimination of benzodiazepines (Doherty, 1991). To avoid prolonged sedation, the dose of benzodiazepine administered to patients with hepatic disease should be modified. Since patients with renal disease exhibit little change in clearance, no dose adjustment is necessary (Esch, 1995).

Other patient populations at increased risk for complications from IV conscious sedation and analgesia include those with chronic cardiac or pulmonary dysfunction. Because chronic obstructive pulmonary disease (COPD) limits respiratory reserve, the respiratory depressive effect of benzodiazepines is exaggerated (Somerson, Husted, & Sicilia, 1995). In patients with congestive heart failure normal doses of benzodiazepines may cause cardiac depression from medullary vasomotor depression (Doherty, 1991). Finally, alcoholic patients and other substance abusers are at risk for having the desire for intoxication stimulated by the use of benzodiazepines in IV conscious sedation (Latham, 1995).

Obese patients who are 30% above their ideal weight are also at increased risk for complications during IV conscious sedation and analgesia. A larger body mass requires a higher cardiac output to perfuse all tissues. An elevated metabolic rate creates more waste production (carbon dioxide) at the cellular level. For excretion of a larger amount of carbon dioxide, a higher rate of ventilation must occur. Therefore these patients may not be able to tolerate a depressed respiratory rate during IV conscious sedation and analgesia. In addition, the risk for aspiration is increased because of abdominal compression of the lungs in the supine position (James, 1996).

When the potential impact of comorbidities is considered and increased vigilance is used during monitoring, older and medically tenuous patients can still safely undergo IV conscious sedation and analgesia. A 1993 prospective study demonstrated that urologic procedures using IV conscious sedation and analgesia could be performed on high-risk patients in an outpatient setting. A total of 7000 patients with significant coronary artery disease, angina, COPD, and asthma were treated with no serious problems. Caregivers believed that a consistent monitoring and treatment approach prevented any major complications (Briggs et al., 1995).

NEUROLOGIC COMPLICATIONS

Oversedation

The RN must recognize that sedation is dose dependent and occurs along a continuum beginning with conscious sedation and analgesia. As the dose of sedation increases, the patient progresses toward general anesthesia (Stanski, 1992). As the level of sedation deepens, hypnosis, motor incoordination, ataxia, and confusion occur. Ultimately the patient becomes obtunded and stuporous and cannot be aroused. As the patient becomes oversedated, he or she becomes flaccid and cannot exhibit any behavioral symptoms of pain. Unfortunately, if the level of analgesia is inadequate, the oversedated patient may still be experiencing pain (Clark, 1994).

Careful assessment and rapid intervention will prevent an overdose. To monitor the patient's level of comfort and consciousness, verbal interaction with the patient should be maintained during the procedure. At no time should the patient lose consciousness. The opioid and the benzodiazepine should both be carefully titrated to the desired end-points of analgesia and sedation. Although it is more time-consuming to administer smaller doses more frequently, larger doses given at less frequent intervals tend to overshoot the goals of IV conscious sedation and analgesia. Oversedation occurs with the accumulation of drug from multiple large doses of medication not cleared quickly enough from the system. In the event that a loss of consciousness occurs, the RN should immediately notify the physician, maintain a patent airway, and anticipate administering reversal agents to antagonize the effects of the benzodiazepines and/or opioids. The use of reversal agents is addressed later in this chapter.

Undersedation

Undersedation can be just as devastating a complication as oversedation. During frightening or uncomfortable procedures patients are under stress both mentally and physically. Mental and physical stress cause the activation of the fight-or-flight response from the autonomic nervous system. This is a defensive reaction that assists the body in physiologically coping with noxious stressors. During the fight-or-flight response, catecholamines are released. Catecholamines increase heart rate, cardiac output, and blood pressure in an attempt to provide more blood flow to vital organs to allow the body to withstand any deleterious assault (Guyton, 1992). During the fight-or-flight response the heart works more vigorously, and myocardial oxygen consumption is increased, potentially causing myocardial ischemia. If sedation is ineffective, the patient will exhibit signs of nervousness and anxiety more than 50% of the time. Additional sedation is beneficial if the patient continues to communicate clearly and succinctly. The patient should be sedated until speech is slightly slurred. However, the patient should still be able to follow all verbal commands (Clark, 1994).

Pain exacerbates anxiety and anxiety exacerbates pain. Therefore, in addition to undersedation, the undertreatment of pain during IV conscious sedation and analgesia can initiate the same detrimental stress response (Halloran & Pohlman, 1995). Additional analgesia is required if the patient verbalizes discomfort, resists, grimaces, or pulls away during the procedure (Clark, 1994).

If the patient can remember over 75% of the procedure, the level of sedation used during IV conscious sedation and analgesia was suboptimal. Patients with this amount of recall usually have a negative perception of the procedure. To minimize the potentially damaging stress response and to attain the amnesic goals of IV conscious sedation and analgesia, undersedation and the undertreatment of pain must be recognized and treated (Clark, 1994).

PARADOXICAL REACTIONS

A small number of patients experience paradoxical reactions to conscious sedation and analgesia. Agitation and dysphoria may occur instead of sedation and relaxation. Although such paradoxical reactions are more common in the pediatric population, adults can also respond in this manner (Walsh, 1995). Case studies involving incoherent shouting and agitation have been reported in adults immediately after the administration of benzodiazepines. After encountering this response, Honan used a reversal agent with his patients and aborted the procedure, whereas Smith continued administering incremental doses of benzodiazepine. Smith reports achieving conscious sedation and analgesia without further complications. In both cases diazepam was used as the sedative, but only Smith used meperidine as the analgesic. Following the procedure only Honan's patients experienced total recall (Smith, 1995; Honan, 1994).

Before the patient's paradoxical reaction is assumed to be a response to a certain medication, other potential causes must be ruled out. Undermedication for pain may be a cause of agitation and restlessness. This may not be recognized in patients unable to verbalize their pain (Agency for Health Care Policy and Research, 1993).

Oversedation can cause hypoventilation, potentially resulting in tissue hypoxia. Cerebral hypoxia or anoxia will initially lead to agitation followed by a decrease in level of consciousness and coma. While the patient is agitated, the RN should protect him/her from injury, ensure a patent airway, and maintain adequate vital signs. While attempting to identify the cause of a paradoxical response to sedation, the RN should check the patient's cardiopulmonary and pain status before assuming that additional sedation will correct the problem. Additional sedation in a hypoxic patient will result in general anesthesia and the need for life support (Doherty, 1991).

PULMONARY COMPLICATIONS

Airway Obstruction

In addition to neurologic complications, sedative-analgesic combinations used during IV conscious sedation and analgesia can also cause a variety of pulmonary disorders. In addition to altering protective reflexes that assist in maintaining a patent airway, benzodiazepines and opioids can produce a loss of submandibular muscle tone. The submandibular muscles provide direct support of the tongue and indirect support of the epiglottis. The tongue may be displaced posteriorly and occlude the airway at the level of the pharynx, and the epiglottis may occlude the airway at the level of the larynx. The tongue, epiglottis, or both can occlude the entrance of the trachea. In the unconscious patient the tongue is the most common cause of airway obstruction. If the airway is not cleared, hypoxia and cardiopulmonary collapse will soon follow (Cummins, 1994).

To identify and treat an obstructed airway, the RN carefully observes chest and abdominal movement for coordination with ventilatory efforts. Movement of air at the nose or mouth area should be verified. With partial airway obstruction the patient may exhibit a weak, ineffective cough, a high-pitched noise while inhaling, uncoordinated attempts at ventilation, and cyanosis. With complete airway obstruction the movement of air is absent. Cyanosis and hypoxia will rapidly result if not treated (Cummins, 1994).

The airway should immediately be restored via the head tilt–chin lift maneuver (Figure 4-1). The goal is to anteriorly displace the mandible. One hand is placed on

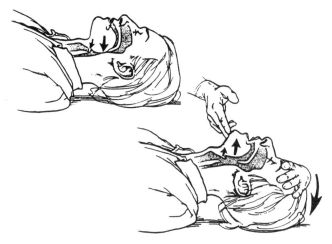

FIGURE 4-1 | Relief of airway obstruction via head tilt–chin lift procedure. (Reproduced with permission. From Cummins, R. [1994]. *Textbook of advanced cardiac life support.* Copyright © American Heart Association.)

the patient's forehead, and pressure is applied to tilt the head back. The fingers of the other hand are placed under the bony part of the jaw and lifted to bring the chin forward, assisting the head in tilting back. In many cases the patient will be able to maintain spontaneous respiration with proper positioning. When airway obstruction persists despite maximal mandibular displacement, insertion of a nasopharyngeal artificial airway may be necessary. However, this device must be used with caution since it might precipitate laryngospasm and vomiting in a semiconscious patient. An oropharyngeal airway should never be used in a semiobtunded patient because of the great risk of laryngospasm. After inserting the airway, the RN should continue to monitor for spontaneous respirations. If spontaneous respirations are absent, artificial positive pressure ventilation should be begun (Cummins, 1994).

Aspiration

Aspiration is the most common cause of death associated with IV conscious sedation and accounts for 1% to 20% of all deaths involving sedation and/or anesthesia. Although complications arising from the aspiration of gastric contents may consist of only bronchospasm, most patients suffer from more serious disorders such as pneumonitis or hypoxia-induced multiorgan failure. Therefore mortality after aspiration is significant, ranging from 5% to 70% (James, 1996). Patients who survive tend to experience prolonged and costly stays in the hospital. The average hospital stay is 21 to 28 days, with the majority of time spent in the intensive care unit (Gibbs & Modell, 1995).

Regurgitation occurs when gastric contents pass from the stomach across the gastroesophageal sphincter into the esophagus and the pharynx. If the larynx is incompetent, gastric contents may be aspirated into the lungs (James, 1996). The likelihood of aspiration is increased with IV conscious sedation and analgesia because protective reflexes, such as the cough and gag reflex, may be impaired or absent with excess sedation (Clark, 1994).

Symptoms of aspiration depend on the extent of pulmonary injury and the material aspirated. Bronchospasm occurs initially because of reflex airway closure. Gastric contents are toxic, causing disruption of the alveolar capillary membrane. A compromised alveolar capillary membrane may result in atelectasis, noncardiogenic pulmonary edema, and even adult respiratory distress syndrome (ARDS). The patient may exhibit all or a few of the following common symptoms: wheezing, crackles, coughing, hypoxia, pulmonary edema, cyanosis, fever, and hyperventilation (Gibbs & Modell, 1995).

Prevention is the best way to address gastric aspiration because the majority of associated complications are severe. Prevention of gastric aspiration begins with the identification of high-risk individuals. The risk of aspiration during a procedure is elevated in any patient undergoing IV conscious sedation and analgesia. This risk escalates for pregnant patients, obese patients, older adult patients, and patients with hiatal hernias or gastroesophageal reflux (James, 1996).

If nausea and vomiting are prevented, the risk for gastric aspiration is reduced. Opioids can induce regurgitation because they stimulate the vomiting center in the medulla. The vomiting center controls the motor impulses required to vomit. Therefore patients receiving benzodiazepines and opioids during IV conscious sedation and analgesia are already at risk for nausea and vomiting. Those at increased risk for nausea and vomiting include children, obese patients, patients with a history of nausea and vomiting associated with sedation, and patients with a history of motion sickness (Nachman, 1993). Reports have also implicated unrelieved pain as a causative factor in postprocedure nausea and vomiting. As the pain was treated, the feeling of nausea subsided (Parnass, 1993). In addition, gastrointestinal secretions and decreased gastrointestinal motility can also contribute to nausea and vomiting (Nachman, 1993). To reduce the incidence of nausea and vomiting, the patient

---

BOX **4-2** *Characteristics of Antiemetics Used During IV Conscious Sedation and Analgesia*

METOCLOPRAMIDE HYDROCHLORIDE (REGLAN)

Action: Accelerates gastric emptying and intestinal transit
Adverse reactions/side effects: Mild sedation (50% of patients), fatigue, restlessness, diarrhea

PROMETHAZINE HYDROCHLORIDE (PHENERGAN)

Action: Acts as an amnesic, antiemetic, antihistamine, and anti–motion-sickness drug; antiemetic action is due to depression of chemoreceptor trigger zone in the medulla
Adverse reactions/side effects: Drowsiness, confusion, restlessness, respiratory depression, blurry vision

DROPERIDOL (INAPSINE)

Action: Antagonizes the emetic actions of narcotics that act on the chemoreceptor trigger zone
Adverse reactions/side effects: Drowsiness, restlessness, hypotension, tachycardia

ONDANSETRON HYDROCHLORIDE (ZOFRAN)

Action: Selectively antagonizes serotonin receptors in the chemoreceptor trigger zone (when serotonin is released, the vomiting reflex is stimulated)
Adverse reactions/side effects: Sedation, headache, dizziness, diarrhea

PROCHLORPERAZINE (COMPAZINE)

Action: Antiemetic action is a result of the suppression of the chemoreceptor trigger zone; weak tranquilizer effect is due to the blockade of postsynaptic dopamine receptors in the brain
Adverse reactions/side effects: Drowsiness, dizziness, extrapyramidal reactions

should have nothing by mouth (NPO) for at least 4 hours before IV conscious sedation and analgesia (and usually the night before) to ensure that the stomach will be empty of food (Maltby, Reid, & Hutchinson, 1988). The American Academy of Pediatrics Committee on Drugs recommends that children remain NPO for no longer than 4 hours before IV conscious sedation and analgesia to avoid dehydration (Kauffman et al., 1992). Antiemetics are most effective when administered before the sedative-analgesic combination. The side effects of most antiemetic drugs are drowsiness and sedation. Therefore unintentional oversedation may result when antiemetics are given with high doses of benzodiazepines and opioids (Tobias, 1993). The RN must be aware of the potential complications that can result from the concurrent use of antiemetics, benzodiazepines, and opioids (Box 4-2).

To prevent aspiration the patient's level of sedation should be vigilantly assessed. This will avert oversedation and the consequent loss of protective airway reflexes. If the patient begins to vomit during the procedure, immediate placement on his/her side and elevation of the head will decrease the risk of aspiration. The airway should immediately be cleared of vomitus with a rigid pharyngeal catheter (Yankauer) and suction (Cummins, 1994).

Immediately after aspiration, the patient may only require the maintenance of a patent airway, oxygen, and observation. Patients with more severe aspiration may require intubation and mechanical ventilation. Therapy may range from the administration of supplemental oxygen to the use of continuous positive airway pressure. Treatment after aspiration is aimed at restoring pulmonary function as rapidly as possible by maintaining an arterial oxygen partial pressure (PaO_2) above 60 mm Hg. Observation and supplemental oxygen therapy to assist the patient in maintaining an adequate PaO_2 may be the only treatment necessary. With more severe aspiration the use of continuous positive airway pressure (CPAP), via a tight-fitting face mask, may be required. The rationale for early use of CPAP is to restore the functional residual capacity and to reduce intrapulmonary shunting, decreasing the incidence of further lung injury. However, if the level of CPAP required for safe oxygenation is greater than 12 to 14 mm Hg, the high pressure found within the face mask may predispose the patient to even more regurgitation and aspiration by forcing open the esophagogastric junction. The patient should be endotracheally intubated if he/she requires high levels of CPAP, has difficulty maintaining a patent airway, or is not alert (Gibbs & Modell, 1995). Early and aggressive treatment of aspiration may minimize secondary complications that may arise, such as infections, abscesses, and fistulas. Although up to 50% of patients suffer from infections after aspiration, prophylactic antibiotics are usually not recommended. Prophylactic antibiotics alter the normal flora of the respiratory tract, rendering the patient susceptible to more resistant and virulent strains of organisms. Antibiotics are begun only after a specific organism has been identified (James, 1996).

Respiratory Insufficiency

Before pulse oximetry and vigilant respiratory monitoring became routine, mishaps resulting from inadequate ventilation were the most common complications observed during conscious and analgesia sedation and/or anesthesia (American Society of Anesthesiology, 1992). Complications caused by respiratory depression were frequent because the respiratory depression was not recognized until it progressed to respiratory arrest, dysrhythmias, or cardiac arrest. When used in combination, benzodiazepines and opioids are synergistic in their respiratory depressant effect. Causes of compromised respiratory function include a direct depression of respiratory drive in response to hypoxia and a diminished ventilatory response to hypercarbia. In addition, a reduction of muscle tone leading to a weaker ventilatory effort may result in a ventilation and perfusion mismatch (Reves, Glass, & Lubarsky, 1995). Respiratory effects caused by benzodiazepines and opioids are dose related. With an overdose the patient can progress from hypoventilation to apnea. The impact on respiratory function is pronounced in patients with a lesser respiratory reserve such as older adults and those with COPD (Gross et al., 1983).

Vigilant physical assessment of the patient's respiratory effort and the use of pulse oximetry allow for the rapid identification and treatment of respiratory compromise. Observe the patient's respiratory rate, pattern, and tidal volume. The patient's breathing should be regular. Thoracic and abdominal ventilatory muscles should be working in coordination to produce deep breaths (10-15 ml/kg). Breath sounds should be clear on auscultation (Stevens & White, 1995). This assessment will identify any muscular difficulties the patient exhibits during ventilation. Hypoventilation may result in hypercapnia since respirations become sluggish and shallow, allowing carbon dioxide to accumulate in the bloodstream. Hypoxia may occur concurrently because the patient is not inspiring enough oxygen to maintain normal tissue oxygenation. Hypoxia and hypercapnia can both cause cell death, depressed mental activity, and a reduced work capacity of the muscles (Guyton, 1992).

Pulse oximetry is an adjunct in monitoring a sedated patient's respiratory status. Since arterial oxygen saturation (SaO_2) is displayed continuously, hypoxia is identified earlier than by physical assessment alone. A study by O'Connor and Jones compared the use of pulse oximetry against clinical observation in the detection of significant desaturation during endoscopy. An SaO_2 indicative of hypoxemia (less than 85%) did not correlate with a change in skin color or vital signs. According to this study, vigilant assessment alone did not detect the beginning of respiratory insufficiency (O'Connor & Jones, 1990). Another study focusing on the use of physical assessment to identify hypoxia demonstrated that an SaO_2 of 80% was the earliest point at which experienced clinicians identified the occurrence of hypoxia (Cohen, Downes, & Raphaely, 1988). Although the following are late signs of inadequate ventilation and oxygenation, they assist the caregiver in identifying severe hypoxia and hypercapnia. Signs and symptoms include a decreased level of consciousness, depressed and shallow respirations, use of accessory muscles, cyanosis (especially in the highly vascular areas such as the lips, nail beds, tip of the nose, and underside of the tongue), diaphoresis, nasal flaring, and agitation (Guyton, 1992).

With the standard use of pulse oximetry, the number of respiratory problems attributed to hypoxia has dramatically decreased (American Society of Anesthesiology, 1992). Early identification and treatment of even a slight decrease in oxygen saturation is now possible with the use of pulse oximetry (Hinzmann, Budden, & Olson, 1992). Respiratory depression can be prevented or minimized by careful titration of benzodiazepines and opioids, with smaller and more frequent doses given on an as-needed basis instead of larger intermittent boluses (Stevens & White, 1995). If the patient becomes hypoxemic, a patent airway is ensured and supplemental oxygen is applied to keep PaO_2 >60 to 70 mm Hg. Depending on the amount of oxygen required, the mode of delivery will vary from the low-flow systems (nasal cannula supplying 24% to 44% inspired fraction of oxygen [FiO_2]) to a face mask providing concentrations of oxygen from 40% to 60% or a face mask with oxygen reservoir where oxygen can be supplied up to 100% (Cummins, 1994). In hypoventilation hypoxia the patient breathing 100% oxygen can intake five times as much oxygen into the alveoli with each respiration as compared with breathing room air (Guyton, 1992).

If the patient becomes apneic, a bag-valve device consisting of a self-inflating bag and a nonrebreathing valve may be required until the patient can be emergently intubated and mechanically ventilated. For adequate ventilation and oxygenation, the caregiver must attain a seal around the patient's face that forces all oxygen into the lungs. The caregiver is positioned near the patient's head. An open airway must be maintained under the mask through the head tilt–chin lift maneuver. The mask is applied to the face while the left hand keeps a tight seal around the face. The bag is compressed with the right hand, and 15 breaths per minute are administered. To ensure proper technique, the chest is observed for rising and falling during ventilation (Cummins, 1994).

CARDIOVASCULAR COMPLICATIONS

Hypotension

Cautious monitoring of the cardiovascular system provides early warning of deleterious side effects that may be caused by drugs used during IV conscious sedation and analgesia. Benzodiazepines and opioids are synergistic in their impact on the cardiovascular system (Reves, Glass, & Lubarsky, 1995). Direct actions on peripheral circulation cause vasodilation with resultant hypotension. With vasodilation, blood pools in the vasculature and is not returned to the myocardium, causing a decrease in cardiac output. The decreased cardiac output may be severe enough to cause cell ischemia and necrosis resulting from an inability to deliver oxygen and nutrients to the tissues. This hypotensive state may be extremely serious in the hypovolemic patient, causing a state of shock. Untreated hypoxia will compound the vasodilatory effects of the drugs and result in a more serious hypotension. Vasodilation occurs in response to hypoxia to increase the blood flow to the tissues and to open more capillaries to increase the surface area for gas exchange. Both responses attempt to augment oxygen delivery to the hypoxic tissues (Durieux & Longnecker, 1996).

In response to hypotension due to vasodilation, the cardiovascular system attempts to compensate with the autonomic nervous system's fight-or-flight response. Endogenous catecholamines such as epinephrine and norepinephrine are released to increase the heart rate and force of contraction. Those patients with cardiovascular disease must be more vigilantly observed because they may not have enough cardiac reserve to mount a response to hypotension (Durieux & Longnecker, 1996).

Careful titration of benzodiazepines and opioids can prevent or minimize any hypotensive effects. Smaller and more frequent doses administered on an as-needed basis, instead of larger intermittent doses of benzodiazepines and opioids, decrease the occurrence of vasodilation. To proactively identify cardiovascular complications, the patient's cardiovascular vital signs should be assessed. The heart rate should be regular. The heart rate and blood pressure should be within normal limits for the patient. Current vital signs should be compared to the patient's baseline. The patient's preprocedure blood pressure might not be representative of an average blood pressure because it might be elevated as a result of anxiety. The patient's peripheral perfusion should be assessed by observing skin color and capillary refill of nail beds. After the procedure the patient should be assisted to first dangle, then sit, then slowly stand to prevent the occurrence of orthostatic hypotension. The patient's blood pressure should be checked in the various positions to ensure hemodynamic stability. If the systolic blood pressure drops by 15 mm Hg or more, the patient should be maintained in the last position until the blood pressure normalizes (Stevens & White, 1995).

If the patient experiences hypotension, he/she should be placed in the Trendelenburg position to redistribute blood from the extremities to the myocardium and thus increase the cardiac output. With more severe and sustained hypotension, fluid therapy must be used to restore effective circulating blood volume. According to the general guidelines regarding the administration of IV conscious sedation and analgesia, an indwelling IV catheter must be prophylactically inserted in all patients. Therefore fluid therapy as well as any emergency drug therapy can be initiated within seconds (Luyk & Ferguson, 1993). Crystalloid solutions such as normal saline or Ringer's lactate are commonly used to treat a hypotensive episode (Clark,

1994). Because fluids may be ineffective in extreme circumstances, vasoactive infusions may also be necessary. Inotropic agents such as dopamine, dobutamine, and epinephrine will increase blood pressure and tissue perfusion by increasing cardiac output, whereas alpha-adrenergic drugs such as norepinephrine and phenylephrine will increase blood pressure by vasoconstricting the peripheral vasculature (Somerson, Husted, & Sicilia, 1995). By knowing the actions and side effects of these emergent drugs, the RN should be able to prevent a cardiac arrest situation (Box 4-3). Supplemental oxygen will increase oxygen delivery to the tissues while the hypotension is being treated. Any hypoxia that is potentially contributing to the hypotension will also be reversed. Endotracheal intubation and mechanical ventilation may be required if the hypotension is severe enough to depress the level of consciousness through inadequate perfusion of the brain (Cummins, 1994).

BOX 4-3 *Vasoactive Drugs for Treatment of Hemodynamic Instability*

DOPAMINE HYDROCHLORIDE (INTROPIN)

Action: Dopamine's actions are dose related; at intermediate doses (2-10 µg/kg/min) contractility and cardiac output are enhanced; at higher doses (>10 µg/kg/min) vasoconstriction occurs, elevating blood pressure

Adverse reactions/side effects: Tachycardia, arrhythmias, hypertension, headache, nausea/vomiting

DOBUTAMINE HYDROCHLORIDE (DOBUTREX)

Action: Enhances contractility and cardiac output; decreases total systemic vascular resistance

Adverse reactions/side effects: Tachycardia, arrhythmias, palpitations, hypotension, headache, nausea/vomiting

EPINEPHRINE HYDROCHLORIDE (ADRENALIN)

Action: Increases contractility, cardiac output, and heart rate; causes arteriolar vasoconstriction, elevating blood pressure

Adverse reactions/side effects: Tachycardia, arrhythmias, cardiac ischemia, angina, anxiety, nervousness, urinary retention, headache, nausea/vomiting

NOREPINEPHRINE BITARTRATE (LEVOPHED)

Action: Elevates blood pressure through powerful vasoconstrictor of arterial vasculature

Adverse reactions/side effects: Hypertension, palpitations, arrhythmias, chest pain, restlessness, anxiety, headache

PHENYLEPHRINE HYDROCHLORIDE (NEO-SYNEPHRINE)

Action: Elevates blood pressure through arteriolar constriction

Adverse reactions/side effects: Tachycardia, palpitations, hypertension, restlessness, anxiety

Myocardial Ischemia

Myocardial ischemia and injury are a result of an oxygen supply-demand mismatch either from a reduction in oxygen supply or from an increase in oxygen demand. Hypoxia leads to inadequate myocardial oxygenation because there is less oxygen in the bloodstream. Tachycardia also reduces oxygen supply to the heart because it decreases the time spent in diastole (the time when the coronary arteries are perfused). Hypotension caused by vasodilation also decreases oxygen supply to the heart because it reduces blood flow through the coronary arteries. In older adults with coronary artery disease, myocardial oxygen consumption can exceed oxygen delivery even with an adequate blood pressure (Stevens & White, 1995). Anything that increases the workload of the myocardium, such as tachycardia and hypertension from pain and anxiety, increases myocardial oxygen demand. Rapid assessment of myocardial oxygen supply and demand is imperative in the prevention of myocardial ischemia and infarction (Roberts & Tinker, 1996).

Chest pain is a symptom of myocardial ischemia and/or infarction. The pain may be described as pressure, tightness, heaviness, aching, crushing, squeezing, burning, viselike, constricting, or suffocating. The substernal area is the usual location of chest pain, but it may also be retrosternal. The pain may radiate to the neck, jaw, teeth, back, shoulders, arms, elbows, and wrists, usually on the left side. The patient may also complain of palpitations from dysrhythmias. While the patient is experiencing chest pain, the electrocardiogram may exhibit ST-segment depression with T-wave inversion, which disappears after the myocardial ischemia subsides. ST-segment elevation may be observed if myocardial injury is occurring (Roberts & Tinker, 1996).

Knowledge regarding a patient's significant cardiac history will assist in preventing myocardial ischemia and infarction. Oxygen delivery to the heart is always compromised in coronary artery disease because of decreased flow of blood through the constricted coronary arteries. Therefore all patients with coronary artery disease will benefit from the prophylactic use of supplemental oxygen (Cummins, 1994). During times of increased myocardial oxygen demand, nitroglycerin can be administered to patients with coronary artery disease. Nitroglycerin can avert the occurrence of a myocardial infarction because it dilates the coronary arteries, increasing blood flow to the heart. It also vasodilates the venous vasculature, decreasing the amount of blood return to the right side of the heart. As the volume returning to the heart is reduced, myocardial workload and oxygen demand are diminished. As oxygen supply and demand are equalized, myocardial ischemia should abate (Roberts & Tinker, 1996).

Dysrhythmias

Ventricular dysrhythmias commonly occur during times of myocardial ischemia and infarction. If not promptly treated, ventricular dysrhythmias will deteriorate into cardiac standstill. The longer that cardiopulmonary compromise persists, the greater the probability of death (Cummins, Ornato, Thies, & Pepe, 1991). The use of electrocardiographic (ECG) monitoring during IV conscious sedation and analgesia allows early identification and treatment of these serious dysrhythmias (Stevens & White, 1995).

An increased frequency of ventricular premature beats (VPBs) (>6 beats/min) and/or the occurrence of multiform VPBs suggests the existence of multiple areas of myocardial ischemia and/or injury (Figure 4-2). If the injury continues, the rhythm may deteriorate into ventricular tachycardia (Figure 4-3) or ventricular fibrillation (Figure 4-4). Ventricular tachycardia is defined as the presence of more than three successive beats of ventricular origin occurring at a rate higher than 100 beats per minute. Untreated ventricular tachycardia degenerates into ventricular fibrillation, where no organized ventricular depolarization exists. At this point the ventricles do not have a cardiac output, and the patient undergoes cardiac arrest (Akhtar, 1995).

For treatment of such life-threatening dysrhythmias, the American Heart Association has developed Advanced Cardiac Life Support (ACLS) Guidelines. These are

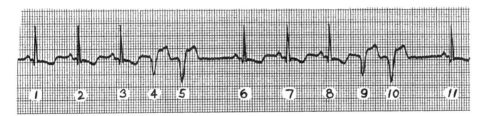

FIGURE 4-2 | Ventricular premature beats. (From Grauer, K., & Cavallaro, D. [1993]. *ACLS certification preparation* [3rd ed., Vol 1]. St. Louis: Mosby.)

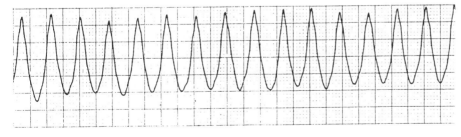

FIGURE 4-3 | Ventricular tachycardia. (From Grauer, K., & Cavallaro, D. [1993]. *ACLS certification preparation* [3rd ed., Vol 1]. St. Louis: Mosby.)

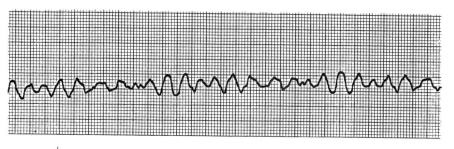

FIGURE 4-4 | Ventricular fibrillation. (From Grauer, K., & Cavallaro, D. [1993]. *ACLS certification preparation* [3rd ed., Vol 1]. St. Louis: Mosby.)

recommendations representing a consensus of experts from a variety of disciplines for emergency cardiac care of patients. According to ACLS guidelines, if the patient's vital signs are stable and the patient is not experiencing chest pain during the ventricular dysrhythmia, a trial of antidysrhythmic therapy may be warranted. Lidocaine, the drug of choice for the suppression of ventricular dysrhythmias, elevates the threshold for the occurrence of ventricular flutter. When using antidysrhythmics such as lidocaine to terminate the dysrhythmias, the RN should identify and treat the underlying cause of the rhythm disturbance (Cummins, 1994).

If the ventricular tachycardia is pulseless or if it deteriorates to ventricular flutter, defibrillation is the most important intervention to be performed immediately because it is the only definitive treatment for pulseless ventricular tachycardia and ventricular flutter. While one caregiver is retrieving the defibrillator, others should be maintaining an airway and administering cardiopulmonary resuscitation (CPR). With defibrillation the goal is to temporarily stop the electrical activity of the heart to allow the natural pacemaker cells to resume activity (Cummins, 1994). Research shows that successive shocks are more important than any drug therapy that delays shocks (Weaver et al., 1990). If patients are not promptly treated, they will deteriorate into asystole within minutes.

Asystole should be treated with CPR, intubation, epinephrine, and atropine. Recently research has supported the use of transcutaneous pacing as an initial response to asystole. Patients who have been in asystole for brief periods have responded to pacing. Simultaneously, the team must attempt to identify and correct the underlying cause of asystole (Bocka, 1989).

Hypoxia and acid-base imbalances, which can occur with IV conscious sedation and analgesia, have also been known to cause pulseless electrical activity (PEA). PEA includes various arrhythmias that do not produce a detectable pulse. In addition to identifying and treating the underlying cause, epinephrine is administered as the drug of choice in treating these serious dysrhythmias (Cummins, 1994).

REVERSAL AGENTS

Although the benzodiazepines and the opioids used in IV conscious sedation and analgesia generally have a proven safety record and are highly effective within a wide therapeutic window, certain instances may require their reversal. Even with close monitoring, the potential exists for overdosing with benzodiazepines and opioids. Deleterious effects such as prolonged sedation, oversedation, airway compromise, and cardiopulmonary depression can result. In addition to treating the complications by the traditional methods noted throughout this chapter, the RN may be required to administer a benzodiazepine or a narcotic receptor antagonist in an attempt to reverse the effects of the benzodiazepine and/or opioid. Unfortunately, reversal agents carry with them the potential for adverse effects. To be able to provide total care for the patient, the RN must understand the side effects as well as the expected actions of these agents (Somerson, Husted, & Sicilia, 1995).

Flumazenil

Flumazenil (Romazicon), synthesized in 1979 by Roche Laboratories, is a reversal agent that competes with benzodiazepines for the same receptor sites. As flumazenil binds with benzodiazepine receptors, benzodiazepines are displaced and their effects are blocked. Depressed level of consciousness, psychomotor impairment, and other cognitive deficits are counteracted. Flumazenil does not consistently reverse benzodiazepine-induced amnesia (Reves, Glass, & Lubarsky, 1995). As flumazenil removes the sedative effects of benzodiazepines, respiratory depression and hypoventilation improve indirectly. Flumazenil has no effect on respiratory depression if it has been induced by opioids (Weinbrum & Geller, 1990).

The onset of flumazenil's actions is evident within 1 to 2 minutes of injection. Within 3 minutes an 80% response is achieved, with the peak effect occurring within 6 to 10 minutes (Roche, 1994). Flumazenil should be titrated by the use of a series of small injections instead of a single large bolus. This enables the caregiver to awaken the patient gradually and minimizes the adverse effects. A dose of 0.2 mg IV is administered over 15 seconds. If the desired level of consciousness has not been achieved within 45 seconds, another dose of 0.2 mg IV should be administered. This pattern should be continued until a maximum dose of 1 mg is reached (Claussen, 1992).

The duration and degree of reversal depends on the amount of flumazenil administered and the plasma concentration of the benzodiazepine (Phillip, Simpson, Hauch, & Mallampati, 1990). In healthy individuals the half-life of flumazenil is 0.8 hours. Since flumazenil is extensively cleared by the liver, its half-life is prolonged to 2.4 hours in patients with severe hepatic disease. The same initial dose of flumazenil should be administered to patients with hepatic dysfunction, but subsequent doses should be reduced in size or frequency. Age, gender, and renal function do not alter the rate of flumazenil clearance (Roche, 1994).

Most benzodiazepines have half-lives that are longer than that of flumazenil. Therefore the potential for resedation exists. As flumazenil is metabolized, sufficient amounts of benzodiazepine are left at the receptor site to cause resedation. Resedation occurs in 3% to 9% of all patients. It is most common in patients who have received high doses of benzodiazepine. After administration of flumazenil, the patient should be monitored for an adequate period (up to 120 minutes) based on the dose and duration of the benzodiazepine used. This will allow the caregiver to identify resedation, respiratory depression, or other residual benzodiazepine effects (Roche, 1994). If resedation occurs, no more than 1 mg IV should be given within a 20-minute period. (To awaken the patient slowly, small doses of 0.2 mg can be administered every 5 minutes.) The maximum dose administered should not exceed 3 mg per hour (Claussen, 1992).

Flumazenil is generally well tolerated, with the most common side effect categorized as transient and mild to moderate in severity (Kasson, 1992). Information regarding specific side effects is listed in Table 4-2. The use of flumazenil has been associated with the occurrence of seizures. Patients at risk for this complication are those who have been administered benzodiazepines for long-term sedation. Patients who are suffering from a serious cyclic antidepressant overdose are also at high risk

TABLE 4-2 *Complications Commonly Associated With Use of Flumazenil*

COMPLICATION	PERCENT
Nausea and vomiting	11
Dizziness	3-9
Injection site pain	
Increased sweating	
Abnormal / blurry vision	
Headache	
Agitation	
Cutaneous	1-3
Fatigue	
Emotional lability	
Paresthesia	
Seizures	
Hypertension	<1
Chest pain	
Arrhythmias (bradycardia, tachycardia)	
Rigors	

Modified from Roche Laboratories (1994). Romazicon (flumazenil) drug insert. Copyright by Hoffman-LaRoche, Inc.

for seizures. Flumazenil is contraindicated in cases of severe cyclic antidepressant poisoning. The patient should remain sedated and mechanically ventilated until signs of antidepressant toxicity have resolved (Roche, 1994).

Respiratory depression and central nervous system depression during IV conscious sedation and analgesia also may be caused by an opiate overdose. Flumazenil will not reverse these effects. The reversal agents naloxone hydrochloride and nalmafene hydrochloride are effective in this situation.

Naloxone

Although the mechanism of action of naloxone hydrochloride (Narcan) is not fully understood, studies suggest that it competes with narcotics for the mu, kappa, and delta receptors. By binding with these receptors, naloxone counteracts the sedation, respiratory depression, analgesia, hypotension, and gastrointestinal stasis produced by opioids (Hoffman & Goldfrank, 1995). Naloxone is a versatile drug and can be administered via IV, intramuscular, intratracheal, or intralingual routes. In emergent situations the IV route is recommended because it has the most rapid onset of action. When naloxone is administered intravenously, the onset of action is detected within 2 minutes (DuPont, 1995).

The dose of naloxone should be titrated according to patient need for reversal of opiate-induced sedation. Initially 0.1 to 0.2 mg IV is administered. This dose is repeated at 2- to 3-minute intervals until the desired level of reversal is gradually achieved. Abrupt reversal of opiate depression has been known to cause tachycardia, hypertension, diaphoresis, nausea, vomiting, seizures, and cardiac arrest. By administering smaller doses at more frequent intervals, the caregiver can control the rate at which the opiate is reversed. Also, larger than necessary doses of naloxone have the potential to completely reverse all analgesic effects, leading to the return of pain (DuPont, 1995).

Naloxone is rapidly metabolized in the liver and is excreted in the urine. Duration of action varies (approximately 45 minutes) according to the route administered and depending on the dose of opiate received. Since naloxone's duration of action is shorter than that of many opiates, resedation may occur. Patients should be observed for an adequate period based on the dose and duration of action of the opiate administered. Repeat doses of naloxone may be required at 1- or 2-hour intervals (DuPont, 1995).

Naloxone does not exhibit any pharmacologic effects in the absence of opiates. When naloxone was appropriately administered for the reversal of postoperative narcotic depression, a study of 813 patients showed that side effects of naloxone were rare (<1%) and were not associated with adverse patient outcomes (Yealy et al., 1990). However, if naloxone is administered to patients who are physically dependent on opiates, the drug may precipitate acute withdrawal symptoms (Hoffman & Goldfrank, 1995). Rare occurrences of hypertension, hypotension, pulmonary edema, and ventricular arrhythmias have been reported. These events occurred in postoperative patients who had a history of preexisting cardiovascular disease or who received medications with similar detrimental cardiovascular effects. Although the complications observed have not been directly attributed to naloxone, caution should still be used with these patient populations (DuPont, 1995).

Nalmafene

Nalmafene hydrochloride (Revex) is also an opioid antagonist that is capable of reversing the unwanted effects of respiratory depression, sedation, and hypotension that opioids may produce. Nalmafene has no effect on complications not caused by opioids. Nalmafene can be administered via the IV, intramuscular, or subcutaneous routes. Onset of action is detected 5 minutes after the initial administration of nalmafene. Administration of an initial dose of 0.25 µg/kg should be followed by 0.25 µg/kg increments every 2 to 5 minutes until the desired degree of reversal is achieved. A total dose greater than 1 µg/kg does not provide any additional benefit (Ohmeda, 1995).

Nalmafene is metabolized by the liver and is excreted by the kidneys. Although nalmafene is excreted more slowly in patients with hepatic and renal dysfunction, no dose adjustment is necessary for a single dose. However, incremental doses should be administered over 60 seconds to minimize the dizziness and hypertension reported in patients with renal failure. Initial nalmafene plasma concentrations are transiently higher in the older adult. No dose adjustment is required since no adverse events have been observed. Partially reversing doses (1 µg/kg) of nalmafene have a 1-hour duration of action, whereas fully reversing doses (1 mg/70 kg) have lasted several hours. Even though nalmafene is the longest acting parenteral opioid antagonist, the potential for resedation still exists. If respiratory depression recurs, the dose of nalmafene again should be titrated to effect to prevent overreversal (recurrence of pain) (Ohmeda, 1995).

As with naloxone, the abrupt reversal of opioid effects with large doses of nalmafene has resulted in the occurrence of tachycardia, hypertension, diaphoresis, nausea, vomiting, seizures, and cardiac arrest. The incidence of adverse effects was greatest in those patients who received more than the recommended dose of nalmafene. In patients with a physical dependence on opioids and patients who have received large doses of opioids for a prolonged period, nalmafene can cause acute withdrawal symptoms. Although nalmafene has been safely used in patients with cardiovascular disease, excessive doses may lead to hypertension, tachycardia, and increased mortality (Ohmeda, 1995).

CONCLUSION

As with any medical therapy, the use of IV conscious sedation and analgesia can result in the occurrence of complications. This chapter reviewed information required for the management of neurologic, pulmonary, and cardiovascular complications associated with the use of IV conscious sedation and analgesia. Also discussed was the use of reversal agents and other medications integral in the treatment of complications. By anticipating and recognizing potential complications, the RN can intervene rapidly to prevent or minimize an adverse clinical outcome.

REFERENCES

Agency for Health Care Policy and Research. (1993). *Acute pain management in adults: Operative procedures. Quick reference guide for clinicians.* Rockville, MD: U.S. Department of Health and Human Services.

Akhtar, M. (1995). Ventricular tachycardia. In M. Crawford (Ed.), *Current diagnosis and treatment in cardiology* (pp. 269-281). Norwalk, CT: Appleton & Lange.

American Nurses Association. (1991). *Position statement on the role of the registered nurse in the management of patients receiving IV conscious sedation for short-term therapeutic, diagnostic, or surgical procedures.* Washington, DC: Author.

American Society of Anesthesiology. (1992). Anesthesia dateline. *Anesthesia Society of America, 1,* 1-3.

Bailey, B., et al. (1990). Frequent hypoxemia and apnea after sedation with midazolam and fentanyl. *Anesthesiology, 73,* 826-830.

Bocka J. (1989). External transcutaneous pacers. *Annals of Emergency Medicine, 18,* 1280-1286.

Briggs, T., et al. (1995). Urological day case surgery in elderly and medically unfit patients using sedoanalgesia: What are the limits? *British Journal of Urology, 75,* 708-711.

Clark, B. (1994). A new approach to assessment and documentation of conscious sedation during endoscopic examinations. *Gastroenterology Nursing, 16*(5), 199-203.

Claussen, D. (1994). Versed administration for IV conscious sedation. *Gastroenterology Nursing, 17*(2), 80-84.

Claussen, D. (1992). Drug forum: Flumazenil. *Gastroenterology Nursing, 14*(5), 263-265.

Cohen, D., Downes, J., & Raphaely, R. (1988). What difference does pulse oximetry make? *Anesthesiology, 68,* 181-185.

Coplans, M., & Curson, I. (1982). Deaths associated with dentistry. *British Dentistry Journal, 153,* 357-360.

Cote, C. (1995). Monitoring guidelines: Do they make a difference? *American Journal of Roentgenology, 165,* 910-912.

Cummins, R. (Ed.). (1994). *Textbook of advanced cardiac life support.* Dallas,TX: American Heart Association.

Cummins, R., Ornato, J., Thies, W., & Pepe, P. (1991). Improving survival from sudden cardiac arrest: The "chain of survival" concept. *Circulation, 83,* 1832-1847.

Daily, E., & Schroeder, J. (1994). *Techniques in bedside hemodynamic monitoring* (5th ed.). St. Louis: Mosby.

Doherty, M. (1991). Benzodiazepine sedation in critically ill patients. *AACN Clinical Issues in Critical Care Nursing, 2*(4), 748-761.

DuPont, (1995). Narcan (naloxone hydrochloride) drug insert. Manati, Puerto Rico: DuPont, Merck Pharmaceuticals, Inc.

Durieux, M., & Longnecker, D. (1996). Failure of the peripheral circulation. In N. Gravenstein & R. Kirby (Eds.), *Complications in anesthesiology.* (2nd ed., pp. 321-333). Philadelphia: Lippincott-Raven Publishers.

Esch, N. (1995). Sedation and pain control in the critically ill patient maintained on continuous neuromuscular blockade. *Critical Care Nursing Quarterly, 18*(2), 85-95.

Fallacaro, M. (1993). A biting commentary on monitored anesthesia care with conscious sedation. *Journal of the American Association of Nurse Anesthetists, 61*(3), 229-232.

Gibbs, C., & Modell, J. (1995). Pulmonary aspiration of gastric contents: Pathophysiology, prevention, and management. In R. Miller (Ed.), *Anesthesia* (pp. 1437-1464). New York: Churchill Livingstone.

Grauer, K., & Cavallaro, D. (1987). *ACLS* (3rd ed.). St. Louis: Mosby.

Gross, J., et al. (1983). Time course of ventilatory depression after thiopental and midazolam in normal subjects and in patients with chronic obstructive pulmonary disease. *Anesthesiology, 58,* 540.

Guyton, (1992). *Human physiology and mechanisms of disease* (5th ed.). Philadelphia: W.B. Saunders.

Halloran, T., & Pohlman, A. (1995). Managing sedation in the critically ill patient. *Critical Care Nurse, 15*(4 Suppl), 1-16.

Hinzmann, C., Budden, P., & Olson, J. (1992). Intravenous conscious sedation use in endoscopy: Does monitoring of oxygen saturation influence timing of nursing interventions? *Gastroenterology Nursing, 15*(9), 6-13.

Hoffman, R., & Goldfrank, L. (1995). The poisoned patient with altered consciousness. *Journal of the American Medical Association, 274*(7), 562-569.

Honan, V. (1994). Paradoxical reaction to midazolam and control with flumazenil. *Gastrointestinal Endoscopy, 40,* 86-88.

James, C. (1996). Pulmonary aspiration of gastric contents. In N. Gravenstein & R. Kirby (eds.), *Complications of anesthesiology* (2nd ed., pp. 175-190). Philadelphia: Lippincott-Raven Publishers.

Jastak, J., & Peskin, R. (1991). Major morbidity or mortality from office anesthetic procedures: A closed claim analysis of 13 cases. *Anesthesia Progress, 38,* 39-44.

Joint Commission on the Accreditation of Healthcare Organizations. (1996). *Comprehensive accreditation manual for hospitals.* Oakbrook Terrace, IL: Author.

Kasson, B. (1992). Flumazenil: A specific benzodiazepine antagonist. *Journal of the Association of Nurse Anesthetists, 60*(5), 472-476.

Kauffman, R., et al. (1992). Guidelines for monitoring and management of pediatric patient during and after sedation for diagnostic and therapeutic procedures. *Pediatrics, 89*(6), 110-114.

Latham, C. (1995). Conscious sedation and the substance abuser. *American Journal of Nursing, 95*(10), 20.

Luyk N., & Ferguson J. (1993). The safe practice of intravenous sedation in dentistry. *New Zealand Dental Journal, 89,* 45-49.

Maltby, J., Reid, C., & Hutchinson, A. (1988). Gastric fluid volume pH in elective patients: Coffee or orange juice versus overnight fast, *Canadian Journal of Anesthesia, 35,* 12-15.

Nachman, J. (1993). Postoperative nausea and vomiting. *Current Reviews in Nursing Anesthesia, 15*(19), 157-164.

O'Connor, K., & Jones, S. (1990). Oxygen desaturation is common and clinically underappreciated during elective endoscopic procedures. *Gastrointestinal Endoscopy, 36,* S2-S4.

Ohmeda Pharmaceuticals. (1995). Revex, nalmafene hydrochloride injection (drug insert). Liberty Corner, NJ: Author.

Parnass, S. (1993). Ambulatory surgical patient priorities. *Post Anesthesia Care Nursing, 28*(3), 531-545.

Phillip, B., Simpson, T., Hauch, M., & Mallampati, S. (1990). Flumazenil reverses sedation after midazolam-induced general anesthesia in ambulatory surgery patients. *Anesthesia & Analgesia, 71,* 371-374.

Proudfoot, J. (1995). Analgesia, anesthesia, and conscious sedation. *Emergency Medicine Clinics of North America, 13*(2), 357-379.

Reves, J., Glass, P., & Lubarsky, D. (1995). Nonbarbiturate intravenous anesthetics. In R. Miller (Ed.), *Anesthesia* (4th ed., pp. 247-259). New York: Churchill Livingstone.

Roberts, S., & Tinker, J. (1996). Perioperative myocardial infarction. In N. Gravenstein & R. Kirby (Eds.), *Complications in anesthesiology* (2nd ed., pp. 335-349). Philadelphia: Lippincott-Raven Publishers.

Roche Laboratories. (1994). Romazicon (flumazenil) drug insert. Nutley, NJ: Hoffman-LaRoche, Inc.

Smith, V. (1995). Paradoxical reactions to diazepam. *Gastrointestinal Endoscopy, 41*(2), 182-183.

Somerson, S., Husted, C., & Sicilia, M. (1995). Insights into conscious sedation. *American Journal of Nursing, 95*(6), 26-33.

Stanski, D. (1992, May). Conscious sedation and its reversal: The pharmacology of conscious sedation and reversal. In D. Fleischer & J. Benjamin (Moderators), *Conscious sedation: Its reversal and monitoring in gastrointestinal endoscopy.* Clinical symposium conducted at the meeting of Society of Gastroenterology Nurses and Associates, San Francisco.

Stevens, M., & White, P. (1995). Monitored anesthesia care. In R. Miller (Ed.), *Anesthesia* (pp. 1465-1480). New York: Churchill Livingstone.

Tobias, J. (1993). Management of minor adverse effects encountered during narcotic administration. *Journal of Post Anesthesia Nursing, 8*(2), 96-100.

Walsh, S. (1995). "Oh no, the patient is six, not sixty!": The pediatric endoscopy patient. *Gastroenterology Nursing, 18*(2), 57-61.

Weaver, W., et al. (1990). Effect of epinephrine and lidocaine therapy on outcome after cardiac arrest due to ventricular fibrillation. *Circulation, 82,* 2027-2034.

Weinbrum, A., & Geller, E. (1990). The respiratory effects of reversing midazolam sedation with flumazenil in the presence or absence of narcotics. *Acta Anaesthesiologica Scandinavica, 92,* 65-70.

Yealy, D., Paris, P., Kaplan, R., Heller, M., & Marini, S. (1990). The safety of prehospital naloxone administration by paramedics. *Annals of Emergency Medicine, 19,* 902-905.

BIBLIOGRAPHY

Association of Operating Room Nurses (1993). Recommended practices: Monitoring the patient receiving IV conscious sedation. *AORN Journal, 57*(4), 978-983.

Brown, K. (1993). Boosting the failing heart with inotropic drugs. *Nursing 93, 23*(4), 34-43.

Shannon, M., & Wilson, B. (1995). *Govoni & Hayes drugs and nursing implications* (8th ed.). Norwalk, CT: Appleton & Lange.

Patient Discharge

A patient who has received conscious sedation and analgesia during a short-term therapeutic, diagnostic, or surgical procedure should be monitored until discharge criteria have been met. Specific criteria for discharge are determined by the physician or are set according to standardized criteria developed by a multidisciplinary team. These criteria assist the physician and the registered nurse (RN) in assessing that the patient is home ready or ready for discharge to an appropriate skilled nursing unit. Documentation should clearly reflect that the patient has met each of the specified criteria.

Following a procedure for which conscious sedation and analgesia has been administered, the patient is usually transferred to a recovery area until determined home ready. The physical location and type of unit used for patient recovery varies and is determined by the institution. Some patients recover on the unit where the procedure was performed (e.g., emergency department), whereas others are transferred to a different area such as short stay. The type of monitoring and criteria for discharge are determined by the procedure performed, the type and amount of medications administered, and the patient's health status.

When care of the patient is transferred from the monitoring RN to a discharge RN or unit RN, the monitoring RN is responsible for providing a concise and detailed report, which should include essential information related to the patient's physiologic and psychologic condition, the sedative and analgesic agents administered, and the procedure (Stein, 1991). This information allows the receiving RN to make a more accurate initial, ongoing, and discharge assessment of the patient.

THE REPORT

The monitoring RN's report may be phoned in or given in person (verbally) to the receiving RN before unit transfer. The report should include, but is not limited to, the following information:

Patient name and age. The RN should know the patient's age and should address the patient with his/her preferred name.

Preexisting medical conditions and preprocedure vital signs. The RN is responsible for total assessment of the patient. Information should include any history of conditions such as respiratory problems, cardiovascular disease, diabetes, hypertension, substance abuse, and posttraumatic stress syndrome. Baseline vital signs should be communicated, and any significant changes should be reported to the physician.

Type of therapeutic, diagnostic, or surgical procedure and physician. Identification of the type of procedure allows the RN to monitor the patient's response to the diagnostic, therapeutic, or surgical intervention. The RN should be aware of the responsible physician in the event that immediate consultation is necessary.

Type of medications, dosage, route, and times. The RN should be informed of all medications administered, total dosage administered, route, and time of last doses. Medications reported include sedative and analgesic agents, reversal agents, and local agents administered during the procedure and any other medications taken the day of the procedure. The RN should be aware of any medications used at home as well as the location of any prescriptions written by the physician following surgery, which should be attached to the chart.

Allergies. The RN should be aware of any allergies to medications, latex, prepping solutions, foods, and environmental allergies.

Intraprocedure monitoring parameters. The RN should be aware of monitoring parameter ranges (e.g., heart rate, respirations, blood pressure, level of consciousness, oxygen saturation, skin condition) and any significant deviation from preprocedure baseline ranges. This information is critical for continuous assessment of the patient throughout the postprocedure period. The RN should notify the physician of any significant changes from preprocedure and intraprocedure monitoring ranges.

Drains, dressings. The RN should be informed of any type of drain, packing, reservoir, and dressing. This information allows the RN to anticipate the type and usual amount of drainage.

Intake and output. The RN should be provided information regarding the amount of intravenous (IV) fluids, irrigation type and amount used, blood loss, and urinary output as appropriate.

Complications. The RN should be apprised of any complications during the procedure, interventions, and patient outcome.

The monitoring RN's report may vary by institution. The preceding listing is minimal information that should be communicated to the RN to allow for an accurate patient assessment for facilitation of quality care.

POSTPROCEDURE ASSESSMENT

The patient is monitored for continued assessment of respiration, circulation, level of consciousness, skin color, and level of voluntary activity. This information should be documented in the patient record. Documentation should reflect continuous evaluation of expected patient outcomes. Multiple scoring systems are used to standardize documentation (e.g., Aldrete & Kroulik, 1970; Aldrete & Wright, 1992; Chung, 1992; Carignan, et al., 1964; Fraulini & Murphy, 1984; Steward, 1975). However, most of these scoring systems were developed for use in phase I of recovery for inpatients recovering from general anesthesia. Generally these scoring systems reflect assessment and documentation of the patient's respirations, circulation, level of consciousness, skin color, and level of voluntary activity.

The Post-Anesthesia Discharge Scoring (PADS) system is specifically designed to measure phase II of recovery and to determine discharge readiness for outpatients (Box 5-1). A score of 2, 1, or 0 is assigned to the main criteria of the PADS system, which include (1) vital signs (i.e., blood pressure, heart rate, respiratory rate, and temperature); (2) activity and mental status; (3) pain, nausea and/or vomiting; (4) surgical bleeding; and (5) intake and output. A score of 9 or 10 indicates that the patient is ready for discharge home. The PADS system has been clinically validated. Because a score of 9 is indicated for discharge, the patient must either void or take fluids. Institutions that have eliminated intake and output from discharge criteria may use another scoring system, such as the Modified Postanesthetic Recovery (PAR) Score for Outpatient's Street Fitness. This scoring system was modified from the Postanesthetic Recovery (PAR) Score that was developed in 1970. Outpatient surgery outdated the PAR scoring system, and in 1992 it was modified to reflect additional assessment factors such as oxygen saturation, dressing, pain management, coordination, urinary output, fasting, and feeding (Box 5-2). Whatever scoring system an institution uses, documentation should reflect objective data supporting the assessment that the patient is stable and suitable for discharge home.

The following Standards of PeriAnesthesia Nursing Practice (1995) are published by the American Society of PeriAnesthesia Nurses (ASPAN) and are applicable to postprocedure management of a patient in phase II, such as a patient receiving IV

BOX 5-1 Post-Anesthesia Discharge Scoring (PADS) System

VITAL SIGNS
2 = Within 20% of preoperative value
1 = 20%-40% of preoperative value
0 = >40% of preoperative value

ACTIVITY AND MENTAL STATUS
2 = Oriented × 3 and a steady gait
1 = Oriented × 3 or a steady gait
0 = Neither

PAIN, NAUSEA, AND/OR VOMITING
2 = Minimal
1 = Moderate, requiring treatment
0 = Severe, requiring treatment

SURGICAL BLEEDING
2 = Minimal
1 = Moderate
0 = Severe

INTAKE AND OUTPUT
2 = Postoperative fluids and void
1 = Postoperative fluids or void
0 = Neither

From Chung F. (1992). New scoring system developed to assess readiness for phase II recovery discharge. *Anesthesia News*, March 1992, pp. 26-27.

BOX 5-2 *Modified Postanesthetic Recovery (PAR) Score for Outpatient's Street Fitness*

ACTIVITY

Able to move four extremities voluntarily on command	2
Able to move two extremities voluntarily on command	1
Able to move no extremities voluntarily on command	0

RESPIRATION

Able to breathe deeply and cough freely	2
Dyspnea or limited breathing	1
Apneic	0

CIRCULATION

BP +20 of preanesthetic level	2
BP +21-49 of preanesthetic level	1
BP +50 of preanesthetic level	0

CONSCIOUSNESS

Fully awake	2
Arousable on calling	1
Not responding	0

O$_2$ SATURATION

Able to maintain O$_2$ saturation >92% on room air	2
Needs O$_2$ inhalation to maintain O$_2$ saturation >90%	1
O$_2$ saturation <90% even with O$_2$ supplement	0

DRESSING

Dry	2
Wet but stationary	1
Wet but growing	0

PAIN

Pain free	2
Mild pain handled by oral meds	1
Pain requiring parenteral meds	0

AMBULATION

Able to stand up and walk straight*	2
Vertigo when erect	1
Dizziness when supine	0

FASTING-FEEDING

Able to drink fluids	2
Nauseated	1
Nausea and vomiting	0

URINE OUTPUT

Has voided	2
Unable to void but comfortable†	1
Unable to void and uncomfortable	0

Data from Aldrete, J., & Wright, A.: *Anesthesia News,* Nov. 1992, pp. 16-17.
*May be substituted by Romberg's test, or picking up 12 clips in one hand.
†Aldrete J. A., Kroulik, D.: A post anesthetic recovery score. (1970). *Anesthesia and Analgesia, 49,* 924-928.

---

conscious sedation and analgesia. Typical goals of nursing care in phase II are summarized in Box 5-3. The patient is encouraged to participate in activities that assist the RN in determining home readiness and appropriateness for discharge.

The ASPAN (1995, pp. 44-45) recommends the following initial, ongoing, and discharge assessment for a patient admitted to a phase II recovery area. These Standards of PeriAnesthesia Nursing Practice (1995) are applicable for any RN managing the recovery of a patient receiving IV conscious sedation and analgesia medications and should be documented (Box 5-4).

BOX **5-3** *Typical Phase II Unit Goals*

- To provide close assessment of and attention to the patient's physical, emotional, and education needs in the postoperative period.
- To provide an environment and personnel who are prepared for emergency interventions at all times.
- To provide family-oriented care that stresses the concept of wellness and acknowledges the integral relationship of the patient and family or other supporting adult.
- To encourage the patient toward as much self-sufficiency as possible, given the type of surgery and anesthesia performed.

- To respect the patient's right to confidentiality, privacy, and respectful, compassionate nursing care.
- To maintain accurate records of patient-related care and environmental preparedness.
- To interact with physicians and other health care providers in a professional manner that results in high-quality patient care.
- To provide patients and families with a resource for questions, comments, and nursing information during their stay and in the immediate period after discharge.
- To offer an environment that encourages the professional growth of nursing personnel.

From Burden, N. (1993). *Ambulatory surgical nursing* (p. 325). Philadelphia: W. B. Saunders.

PATIENT DISCHARGE

The discharge planning process begins when the decision to perform a procedure is made by the patient and physician. The goal is to provide for an organized plan of care based on the patient's needs and health status. The discharge planning process should be responsive to the patient, physicians, and RNs involved in the management of the patient's care. Most patients receiving conscious sedation and analgesia are undergoing a procedure that is relatively short in duration. In establishing a discharge plan for the patient, there must be clear discharge criteria to determine that the patient can safely recover at home.

The Joint Commission on Accreditation of Healthcare Organizations (1996) has developed anesthesia care standards applicable to the patient receiving IV conscious sedation and analgesia. These are excerpted as follows:

> TX.2.4 The patient's postprocedure status is assessed on admission to and before discharge from the postanesthesia recovery area.
> TX.2.4.1 Patients are discharged by qualified licensed independent practitioner or according to criteria approved by the medical staff.

Most institutions have developed specific written criteria for discharge that have been approved by the medical and surgical staff to ensure that the same standard of care is being provided to all patients. Although the physician is ultimately responsible for patient discharge, it is usually the RN who is responsible for determining

INITIAL ASSESSMENT: PHASE II

Initial assessment should include documentation of the following:

1. Integration of data received at transfer of care
2. Vital signs
   a. Respiratory rate and status
   b. Blood pressure
   c. Pulse
   d. Temperature
3. Level of consciousness
4. Position of patient
5. Patient safety needs
6. Condition and color of skin
7. Neurovascular assessment as applicable
8. Condition of dressings, drains, and tubes as applicable
9. Muscular response and strength
10. Fluid therapy, location of lines, condition of IV sites and securement type, and amount of fluid infusing
11. Level of physical and emotional comfort
12. Numerical score if used

ONGOING ASSESSMENT: PHASE II

Ongoing patient care and assessment should include but not be limited to the following:

1. Identification of patient and name family normally uses
2. Monitor, maintain, and/or improve respiratory function
3. Monitor, maintain, and/or improve circulatory function
4. Promote and maintain physical and emotional comfort
5. Monitor surgical site
6. Interpret and document data obtained during assessment
7. Administer analgesics as necessary and record results
8. Administer other medication as ordered and record results
9. Provide maximum degree of privacy
10. Provide for safety
11. Provide for confidentiality of information and records
12. Encourage fluids by mouth
13. Ambulate with assistance
14. Position patient gradually from supine to Fowler's position
15. Ask patient to urinate prior to discharge
16. Review discharge planning with patient, family/accompanying responsible adult as appropriate; provide written home care instructions
17. Provide follow-up for extended care as indicated; next day follow-up call is recommended to evaluate status

DISCHARGE ASSESSMENT: PHASE II

Current assessment data are collected and recorded to evaluate the patient's status for discharge to home:

1. Adequate respiratory function
2. Stability of vital signs, including temperature
3. Level of consciousness and muscular strength
4. Ability to ambulate consistent with developmental age level
5. Ability to swallow oral fluids, cough, or demonstrate gag reflex
6. Ability to retain oral fluid
7. Skin color and condition
8. Pain minimal
9. Adequate neurovascular status of operative extremity
10. Patient and home care provider understands all home instructions
11. Written discharge instructions given to patient/accompanying responsible adult
12. Concur with prearrangements for safe transportation home
13. Provide additional resource to contact if any problems arise

that the patient has met the standardized discharge criteria and that it is reasonable to discharge the patient.

The following parameters for discharge are frequently used to assess readiness for discharge and assist the RN in determining that the patient has returned to a safe physiologic level: stable vital signs, level of consciousness, mobility, airway patency, intact protective reflexes, skin color and condition, condition of dressing and surgical site, absence of protracted vomiting, and ability to urinate (Association of Operating Room Nurses, 1996, p. 208). Table 5-1 identifies typical criteria for common discharge parameters. If the patient fails to meet the identified discharge criteria, the RN should notify the physician and document appropriate interventions as indicated.

DISCHARGE TEACHING AND INSTRUCTIONS

Most patients receiving IV conscious sedation and analgesia are in the institutional setting for a very short time and are discharged home with a responsible escort to continue their recovery. Because the medications administered may result in drowsiness and amnesia, discharge instructions should be explained to both patient and escort. General discharge instructions include basic information such as medications (including scheduled medications, prescribed medications with names, purpose, route, dosage, frequency, duration, and significant or expected side effects); dietary regime; activity and limitations as appropriate; instructions related to postprocedure care; signs/symptoms related to care that may require medical attention; emergency numbers and physician's number; expected follow-up care with the physician; instructions regarding driving limitations; and appropriate referral sources for continuing care needs. Postprocedure instructions may be specific to the type of procedure and possible complications (Figure 5-1).

Information should be documented to reflect patient and escort understanding of discharge instructions (e.g., patient and escort complete successful return demonstration of emptying a drain). A copy should be given to the patient, and a copy should be retained as part of the patient record. Griffith and McLaughlin (1991, p. 56) reported three recurrent reasons that patients gave for failing to seek medical attention for a significant change of symptoms after discharge: (1) not knowing what to look for, (2) not knowing the significance of what he/she subsequently found, and (3) not knowing what he/she was supposed to do or whom to contact.

POSTPROCEDURE PHONE CALL

In some areas the accepted standard of care is a postprocedure phone call (Burden, 1994). This phone call is usually made within 24 hours after the procedure. This allows the RN to assess the patient's health status and determine any immediate needs the patient may have. The patient should be informed of the postprocedure phone call during discharge teaching. Specifically, the patient should be told that once he/she is at home to write down any questions he/she would like to

TABLE 5-1 *Discharge Criteria: Areas of Concern*

DISCHARGE PARAMETER	TYPICAL CRITERIA	COMMENTS
Vital signs	Stable for 30-60 min prior to discharge; no respiratory distress	Requires that more than one set of vital signs is taken and compared with the patient's preoperative normal vital signs
Level of consciousness	Conscious, oriented to surroundings	Level of sedation more difficult to identify—often depends on the quality of adult supervision the patient will have at home
Nourishment and hydration	Able to tolerate and maintain oral fluids	Whether this is actually necessary for healthy adults is controversial; of special concern if patient is elderly, young, or debilitated or if patient has had extensive procedure
Comfort	Comfortable with use of oral analgesics or none; minimal nausea or vomiting	Total freedom from discomfort is not realistic, but the patient should not be discharged with acute symptoms; concern for comfort related to length of ride home and ability to obtain prescription medications
Activity	Able to walk and dress self	If appropriate to patient's preoperative status and to the type of procedure; ensure ability to use crutches, walker PRN; assess patient walking prior to discharge to identify problems such as hypotension or fainting
Surgical site	No untoward symptoms or bleeding; drainage appropriate for procedure; dressing secure; extremity circulation adequate	Patient should understand normal and abnormal parameters and how to check circulation
Instructions	Patient and family or responsible adult should be given verbal and written instructions	Have both sign copy to retain on medical record; individualize for each patient
Responsible adult supervision	Patient to be discharged with responsible adult to drive and remain with patient for 24 hr After local anesthesia without sedation, physician may discharge patient without supervision	Facility should set policies of what is minimum acceptable adult companionship (taxi driver? hospital van driver? minor?) and what actions nurse should take if patient desires to leave against medical advice

From Burden, N. (1994). Post anesthesia care of the ambulatory surgical patient. In C. B. Drain, *The post anesthesia care unit: A critical care approach to post anesthesia nursing* (3rd ed.). Philadelphia: W. B. Saunders.

Lowery A. Woodall, Sr.
OUTPATIENT SURGERY FACILITY
A Division of Forrest General Hospital

POST INSTRUCTIONS FOR LOCAL ANESTHESIA WITH SEDATION

The medication or sedation which was used to calm you will be acting in your body for the next 24 hours, so you might feel a little sleepy. This feeling will slowly wear off. Because the medicine or sedation is still in your system, for the next twenty-four (24) hours, the adult patient:

SHOULD NOT -- Drive a car, operate machinery or power tools.
SHOULD NOT -- Drink any alcoholic beverages (not even beer).
SHOULD NOT -- Make any important decisions (such as sign important papers).

PAIN:
You may have some pain. A prescription for pain may be given by your doctor. This should be taken as directed on the label. If your doctor does not prescribe any pain meds, you may take non-prescription medication, which can be purchased at your drugstore.

DIET:
You may resume your normal diet when you arrive home, unless you are instructed otherwise by your doctor.

ACTIVITY LEVEL:
We strongly suggest you have a responsible adult with you the rest of today and also during the night for your protection and safety. Rest the remainder of today and tonight.

ADDITIONAL INSTRUCTIONS:_____

_____
_____
_____
_____

See Dr. _____ on _____ at _____ in his office.

If you have any questions or concerns, call Dr. _____ at phone _____.

If you are unable to reach him/her or his/her partner, call or come to the Forrest General Hospital Emergency Department at 288-2100.

The information/instructions above have been discussed with and a copy given to me or a significant other who demonstrates an adequate level of understanding and will give these instructions for care to the individual responsible for my care.

_____   _____
Patient/Significant Other   Physician/Nurse

_____ AM _____ PM
Date/Time   Revised 2/6/95
                                                             FGH 211020

FIGURE 5-1 | Post instructions for local anesthesia and sedation. (Courtesy Forrest General Hospital, Hattiesburg, MA.)

discuss during the call. The RN should document any signs and symptoms on the patient chart. Any follow-up, such as immediate referral of the patient to the attending physician and calling the physician with a direct report, also needs to be documented. The postprocedure phone call conveys a positive message to the patient that the health care providers are truly interested in the individual's follow-up care and leads to positive patient satisfaction.

CONCLUSION

The manner in which a patient is discharged is determined by institution policy and procedure. RNs should fully understand their role in the discharge process. Written discharge instructions should be given to the patient, and accurate documentation should be done to reflect the patient's achievement of discharge criteria. The overall goal of well-established discharge criteria is to ensure that the patient has adequately recovered from the effects of the procedure and the medications administered to achieve a state of conscious sedation and analgesia and may safely continue recovery at home.

REFERENCES

Aldrete, J. A., & Kroulik, D. (1970). A post anesthesia recovery score. *Anesthesia and Analgesia, 49*, p. 924.

Aldrete, J., & Wright, A. (1992). Post anesthesia scores. *Anesthesia News,* Nov. 1992, pp. 16-17.

American Society of PeriAnesthesia Nurses. (1995). Resource 7: Preanesthesia, postanesthesia—data required for initial, ongoing, and discharge assessment. In *Standards of perianesthesia nursing practice* (pp. 44-45). Thorofare, NJ: Author.

Association of Operating Room Nurses. (1996). Recommended practices: IV conscious sedation. In *AORN standards and recommended practices* (pp. 205-210). Denver: Author.

Burden, N. (1994). Post anesthesia care of the ambulatory surgical patient. In C. B. Drain (Ed.), *The post anesthesia care unit: A critical care approach to post anesthesia nursing* (3rd ed., pp. 506-516). Philadelphia: W. B. Saunders.

Carignan, G., Keeri-Szanto, M., & Lavellie, J. P. (1964). Postanesthetic scoring system. *Anesthesiology, 25,* 396.

Chung F. (1992). New scoring system developed to assess readiness for phase II recovery discharge. *Anesthesia News,* March 1992, 26-27.

Fraulini, K. E., & Murphy, P. (1984). R.E.A.C.T. A new system for measuring postanesthesia recovery. *Nursing 84, 14*(4), 101-102.

Griffith, J. L., & McLaughlin, S. H. (1991). Legal implications. In B. V. Wetchler (Ed.), *Anesthesia for ambulatory surgery* (2nd ed., p. 56). Philadelphia: J. B. Lippincott.

Stein, R. (1991). The importance of communication between the anesthesiologist and the postanesthesia care unit nurse. *Journal of Post Anesthesia Nursing, 6*(4), 279-281.

Steward D. J. (1975). A simplified scoring system for the post-operative recovery room. *Canadian Anaesthetists Society Journal, 22,* 111.

Institution Policy and Guideline Development: Standard of Care

The administration of conscious sedation and analgesia is a common practice among settings throughout an institution, including the various diagnostic laboratories and departments such as radiology, emergency, surgical services, endoscopy, special procedures, cardiac catheterization, electrophysiology, and others. In the past each department acted independently to determine the standard of care delivered to its patients receiving conscious sedation and analgesia. Today, largely because of the Joint Commission on Accreditation of Healthcare Organizations (JCAHO), institutions now have in place or in development a single standard of care for patients receiving conscious sedation (with or without analgesia) that is consistent institution-wide.

According to the JCAHO (Same-Day Surgery, 1995, p. 122), the anesthesia standards apply to "all use of conscious sedation." Conscious sedation and analgesia is viewed as occurring on a continuum, and it is not possible to predict how a patient who is receiving conscious sedation and analgesia will respond. Because of this, most institutions have developed a single standard of care that is multidisciplinary and addresses protocols that are specific to providing uniform care for any patient receiving conscious sedation and analgesia at the respective institution.

The *1996 Comprehensive Accreditation Manual for Hospitals* standards related to anesthesia care state that:

> The standards for anesthesia care apply when patients in any setting, receive, for any purpose, by any route, (1) general, spinal, or other major regional anesthesia (2) sedation (with or without analgesia) which, in the manner used, may be reasonably expected to result in the loss of protective reflexes (p. 153). ["Loss of protective reflexes" is defined as the inability to handle secretions without aspiration or to maintain a patent airway independently.]

An appropriate standard of care should be developed that addresses care of patients who are at risk for loss of protective reflexes. The JCAHO (1996, p. 153) states that the standard of care for those patients at risk should be developed, should be consistent with professional standards, and should address the following:

- Sufficient qualified personnel present to perform the procedure and to monitor the patient (see TX.2-TX.2.2, LD.2.7 and LD.2.9, and HR.1 and HR.2)

- Appropriate equipment for care and resuscitation (see LD.1.3.2 and EC.2.1.3)
- Appropriate monitoring of vital signs: heart and respiratory rates and oxygenation (see TX.1, TX.2-TX.2.2, TX.3-TX.3.9, and TX.5-TX.5.4)
- Documentation of care (see IM.7.3 - IM.7.4)
- Monitoring of outcomes (see the "Leadership" chapter and PI.3.1-PI.3.2.7)

In addition, the standard of care should include required patient assessment parameters, patient documentation, patient discharge criteria, and educational expectations for nonanesthesia health care providers administering conscious sedation and analgesia in an institution (Holland, 1995).

PROCESS FOR DEVELOPING A SINGLE STANDARD OF CARE

Policies and procedures, standards of care, and critical pathways are all elements used in the process for developing the type of care provided to any patient of an institution who is receiving conscious sedation and analgesia during a short-term diagnostic, therapeutic, or surgical procedure. A single institution-wide standard of care may also assist in measuring patient outcomes, patient satisfaction, and quality of care.

Step 1: Selection of Team Members

Most institutions have in place a standard of care for the administration of conscious sedation and analgesia (Figure 6-1). When it becomes necessary to revise the existing standard of care, team member selection is critical. The person selected to chair the project team should have a proven record as a leader and the ability to move a group forward. It is helpful if the chairperson and other members of the project team are well respected among their peers and are knowledgeable and experienced in the administration of conscious sedation and analgesia. Familiarity with national guidelines and recommendations is desirable.

Some institutions report that revisions to the standard of care for the administration of conscious sedation and analgesia have taken years to make or have not occurred at all because of the turf battles that occur among departments. Therefore the leader must stay focused on the overall goal of the institution-wide standard of care, that is, to deliver safe, high-quality patient care. This individual may guide the group through the process of evaluating the existing standard of care by asking:

- Are we keeping our practices current and correct?
- What practices do the national nursing and medical associations recommend, and what is the local practice?
- Are any recommendations currently not being practiced at the local level?
- Can these be incorporated into the current standard of care?
- Are we measuring quality of care and its improvement?

Any data that have been collected should be analyzed, and plans for improvement should be discussed.

Text continued on p. 113

HARRIS COUNTY HOSPITAL DISTRICT			STATE NO:	4225
PREPARED BY: Special Care Committee	APPROVED BY: *LJM*	ISSUED BY: Medical Board	TITLE: **INTRAVENOUS** **CONSCIOUS SEDATION**	
DATE: June 1995		PAGE 1 OF 4		
PAVILION(S): DISTRICT WIDE			DEPARTMENT(S): DISTRICT WIDE	

PURPOSE

To delineate the practice for the safe and effective administration of conscious sedation in the absence of an Anesthesiologist or Certified Registered Nurse Anesthetist (CRNA).

To provide guidelines for the administration of conscious sedation for diagnostic/therapeutic procedures other than maintenance of endotracheal intubation in the Emergency/Critical Care Units or analgesia for labor and delivery.

DEFINITION

ANESTHESIA

The administration (in any setting, by any route, or for any purpose) of general, spinal, or other major regional anesthesia or sedation (with or without analgesia) for which there is a reasonable expectation that, in the manner used, the sedation/analgesia will result in the loss of protective reflexes for a significant percentage of a group of patients. (JCAHO)

CONSCIOUS SEDATION

A medically controlled state of depressed consciousness is characterized by:

- Protective reflexes that are maintained
- Patent airway independently maintained and continuously intact
- Appropriate response to physical stimulation or verbal command

DEEP SEDATION

A medically controlled state of depressed consciousness or unconsciousness is characterized by:

- Patient not easily aroused
- Partial or complete loss of protective reflexes
- Inability to maintain a patent airway independently
- Absence of purposeful response to physical stimulation or verbal command

PRACTITIONERS

MD   Medical Doctor
DO   Doctor of Osteopathy
DDS   Doctor of Dental Science
APN   Advanced Practice Nurse (i.e., Midwife, Nurse Practitioner, Clinical Specialist)

POLICY

1. Conscious sedation may be administered by:
   - **Physicians/dentists** credentialed by their respective Department and the Medical Staff of Harris County Hospital District (HCHD) to perform such procedures and who have documented competency in airway management
   - **Advanced Practice Nurses** credentialed by their respective Department and/or Harris County Hospital District (HCHD) Nursing Services to perform such procedures and who have documented competency in airway management
   - **Registered Nurses** under the <u>direct supervision</u> of an appropriately credentialed physician/dentist, who have successfully demonstrated competency as defined by Harris County Hospital District (HCHD) Nursing Services

FIGURE 6-1 | Sample standard of care for administration of conscious sedation. (Courtesy Harris County Hospital District.)

Continued

2. **Informed Consent** (HCHD 6384) shall be obtained <u>prior</u> to the administration of conscious sedation for patients who are undergoing non-emergency procedures.
3. An Emergency Supply Cart shall be present throughout conscious sedation with appropriate age- and size-dependent airway resuscitation equipment.
4. A registered nurse shall be responsible for monitoring and assessing the patient throughout conscious sedation.
   - The nurse MUST have no responsibilities that would leave the patient unattended or compromise continuous monitoring.
   - Additional nursing or technical support personnel shall assist the physician/dentist with diagnostic/therapeutic procedures that are complicated either by the severity of the patient's illness and/or the complex technical requirements associated with advanced diagnostic/therapeutic procedures.
5. An **Anesthetic Evaluation** form (HCHD 6415) shall be completed <u>prior</u> to non-emergency conscious sedation.
   - If the evaluation is performed by a non-Advanced Practice Nurse (APN), the responsible physician/dentist **MUST** review and countersign the **Anesthetic Evaluation** form (HCHD 6415), which acknowledges that the patient is an appropriate candidate for anesthesia.
6. **INTRAVASCULAR ACCESS** for conscious sedation:
   - <u>**CHILDREN**</u> $\geq$ 6 years of age shall have an established access line <u>prior</u> to conscious sedation.
   - <u>**CHILDREN**</u> $\leq$ 6 years of age at the discretion of the physician/dentist may receive <u>conscious</u> sedation <u>without</u> intravascular access.
   - **ADULTS and CHILDREN** shall have an established access line <u>prior</u> to <u>deep</u> sedation.
7. Vital signs shall be recorded every five (5) minutes <u>during</u> conscious sedation and documented on the **Intravenous Conscious Sedation Assessment** form (HCHD 7139). Monitoring shall include:
   - EKG with oscilloscopic display
   - Blood pressure by non-invasive automated blood pressure
   - Oxygen saturation (SpO_2) with display

Following the conscious sedation, the patient shall be observed in the Post Anesthesia Care Unit (PACU) or in a comparably equipped and staffed recovery area. Vital signs shall be monitored every 15-minutes x4; every 30-minutes x2; and every hour x4 or until such time that the patient meets discharge criteria.

Discharge shall be based on a **Post Anesthesia Recovery Score** (PAR Score).
   - Patients being transferred to a non-critical care unit MUST have a **PAR Score** of $\geq$ **8.**
   - Patients being discharged to home MUST have a TOTAL **PAR Score** of $\geq$ **16.**
8. The physician/dentist, or advanced practice nurse (APN), shall be responsible for assessment for discharge post-conscious sedation. Documentation on the **Anesthetic Evaluation** form (HCHD 6415) should include the presence or absence of conscious sedation–related complications, condition and disposition of the patient.
9. Each department through its established performance improvement programs shall be responsible for monitoring the appropriateness of care during conscious sedation.

PROCEDURE RESPONSIBLE PARTY	ACTION
	PRE-PROCEDURE STAGE
MD, DO, DDS	1. Assesses the patient.
	2. Explains diagnostic/therapeutic procedure(s) and medications to be administered to patient/family.
	3. Obtains **Informed Consent.**
MD, DO, DDS, APN	1. Measures and records baseline vital signs.
	2. Completes the **Anesthetic Evaluation** form (HCHD 6415) to include:
	• History & Physical
	• ASA Score

FIGURE 6-1 cont'd | Sample standard of care for administration of conscious sedation.

- Previous anesthetics and complications
- Operation/Procedure to be performed
- Date/Time of last oral intake
- Allergies
- Current laboratory results
- Current medications
- Diagnosis
- Anesthesia Plan

MD, DO, DDS, APN, RN	1. Establishes/verifies patency of intravenous access.
	2. Prepares equipment/supplies.
	3. Notifies appropriate Medical/Dental personnel of any medical record deficiencies (i.e., H&P, Consents, Lab, etc.) when conscious sedation is being administered.
	4. Completes **Intravenous Conscious Sedation Assessment** form (HCHD 7139) to include: **(Page 1 of Form)** (see Figure 6-3)
	   • Baseline Vital Signs
	   • Psychosocial Assessment
	   • Physical Assessment
	   • Medical/Anesthesia History
	   • Patient Education of Procedure

INTRA-PROCEDURE STAGE
(Page 2 of Form) (see Figure 6-3)

MD, DO, DDS, APN, RN	1. Assures the presence of appropriately equipped Emergency Supply Cart.
	2. Verifies function of oxygen system if appropriate.
	3. Verifies presence of <u>completed</u> **Informed Consent** (HCHD 6384) form.
	4. Assesses patency of intravenous access if appropriate.
	5. Completes **Intravenous Conscious Sedation Assessment** (HCHD 7139):
	   • Vital signs every 5 minutes
	   • Drug/agents, amount, and times of administration
	   • IVF/blood & blood components, amount, and times of administration
	   • Intake/Output
	   • Agents/Techniques used
	   • Unusual events
	   • Condition of the patient at the conclusion of conscious sedation

MD, DO, DDS, APN	1. Performs diagnostic/therapeutic procedure. 2. Documents diagnostic/therapeutic procedure and any pertinent information. 3. Assesses stability for transfer if recovery occurs elsewhere. 4. Writes order for transfer if applicable.

POST-PROCEDURE STAGE
(Page 3 of Form) (see Figure 6-3)

MD, DO, DDS, APN, RN	1. Completes **Intravenous Conscious Sedation Assessment** form (HCHD 7139) to include:
	   • Vital signs:
	      • Every 15-minutes x4
	      • Every 30-minutes x2
	      • Every hour x4.
	   • Drug/agents, amount, and times of administration

FIGURE 6-1 cont'd | Sample standard of care for administration of conscious sedation.
Continued

	• IVF/blood & blood components, amount, and times of administration
	• Intake/Output
	• Diagnostic studies
	• Unusual events
	2. Assesses for discharge per PAR Score
	• ≥ 8 Par Score - Non-critical Care unit
	• ≥ 16 Par Score - Home
	3. Provides post-diagnostic/therapeutic procedure education to patient/family.
MD, DO, DDS, APN	1. Evaluates for discharge/transfer to include:
	• Airway/breathing patency
	• Hemodynamic stability
	• Level of Consciousness
	2. Documents on **Anesthesia Evaluation** form (HCHD 6415):
	• Presence or absence of complications during/post conscious sedation
	• Condition
	• Disposition
	3. Writes order for discharge.

PERFORMANCE IMPROVEMENT

Medical/Nursing	1. Conducts peer review.
	2. Communicates findings.
	3. Develops corrective action plan as indicated.

REVIEWED/APPROVED BY

06/95	Medical Board
06/95	Medical Executive Committees, LBJGH/BTGH
05/95	HCHD Policy & Procedure Committee
06/94	HCHD Policy & Procedure Committee
06/94	Nursing Vice-President Conference
06/94	Operative/Invasive Committee
05/94	Medical Board
05/94	Medical Executive Committees, LBJGH/BTGH

REFERENCES

American Academy of Pediatrics, Guidelines for Monitoring and Management of Pediatric Patients During and After Sedation for Diagnostic and Therapeutic Procedures, Pediatrics, Vol. 89, No. 6, June 1992.

AORN, Recommended Practices for Monitoring the Patient Receiving Intravenous Conscious Sedation, 1993.

JCAHO, Operative and Other Invasive Procedures, Accreditation Manual for Hospitals: Volume II, Scoring Guidelines, 1993, 4.

Neff, J.A., Patient Care Guidelines: Conscious Sedation, Journal of Emergency Nursing, Vol. 18, No. 2, April 1992, 165-167.

Society of Gastroenterology Nurses and Associations, Inc., Nursing Care of the Patient Receiving Conscious Sedation in the Gastrointestinal Endoscopy Setting, 1991.

Texas Board of Nurse Examiners Policies and Procedures, Administration of IV Conscious Sedation by the Registered Nurse, Position Statement 15.18, 1992.

FIGURE 6-1 cont'd | Sample standard of care for administration of conscious sedation.

Step 2: Evaluation of Nationally Endorsed Position Statements, Recommended Practices, and Guidelines

The project team should review available nationally endorsed position statements, recommended practices, and guidelines on the administration of conscious sedation and analgesia (see Chapter 1). Each should be evaluated to determine recommended practices versus actual practices of the institution. Do actual practices vary from national recommendations? If an institution has a practice that differs from national nursing and medical association recommendations, is there any documentation in the literature or other sources to provide support for the local practice? If the project team decides to follow local practice versus the national recommendation, the reasons should be justified, supported, and documented. A plan for monitoring and evaluating patient outcome should be identified (Figure 6-2).

The project team members should review any patient teaching pamphlets (which may be distributed), standardized patient documentation form or flow chart used for documenting the administration of conscious sedation and analgesia (Figure 6-3), standardized discharge criteria, required patient assessments, patient education instruction, and informed consent as appropriate.

Step 3: Determining Policy Format

Each institution should have a designated format for developing policy and procedures, protocols, and standard of care. The following benchmarks could be included in any existing protocol:

Scope of practice. This section should identify the intended health care provider of the protocol. For example, "This protocol applies to all registered nurses at the University Medical Center."

Definition of conscious sedation and analgesia. A concise and well-defined definition should be included to assist in determining appropriate patient populations. The most widely accepted definition from the literature is:

> Intravenous conscious sedation is produced by the administration of pharmacologic agents. A patient under conscious sedation has a depressed level of consciousness, but retains the ability to independently and continuously maintain a patent airway and respond appropriately to physical stimulation and/or verbal command (ANA, 1991).

Purpose. This section should describe the intent of the protocol, for example: The purpose of this protocol is the identify guidelines for the administration of conscious sedation and analgesia to ensure that care throughout the institution is provided by health care providers authorized to do so. Conscious sedation and analgesia may be administered during a short-term diagnostic, therapeutic, or surgical procedure to decrease patient anxiety and discomfort.

Implementation. This section should include necessary supplies and equipment, assessment and monitoring parameters, medication guidelines, discharge criteria, and documentation requirements. *Text continued on p. 119*

CONSCIOUS SEDATION
QUALITY IMPROVEMENT MONITORING AND EVALUATION

POLICY

A. Each department/unit where conscious IV sedation is administered will monitor compliance with predetermined indicators on a continuous basis.

B. A 10% sample size will be utilized.

C. Any fall-outs will be evaluated for cause. (Target: 100%)

D. Data collection frequency is at the discretion of the department/unit. Concurrent data collection is recommended.

E. Data should be included with department/unit quarterly reports and be submitted to the Center for Quality Improvement for aggregation and analysis.

F. Physician-related issues should be referred to the appropriate Medical Director or Chairman.

G. Opportunities for improvement should be corrected as quickly as possible.

H. Data Collection Form:

QUALITY IMPROVEMENT MONITORING DATA COLLECTION FORM
CONSCIOUS SEDATION

UNIT/DEPT: _____ DATE:_____

INDICATORS	YES	NO	COMMENTS
1. Were the preprocedural vital signs documented? (BP, P, RR, T, SaO_2)			
2. Were the sedatives &/or narcotics administered by a licensed nurse or physician?			
3. Was the patient monitored by staff qualified by P/P criteria?			
4. Were the vital signs documented per policy during the procedure?			
5. Were significant changes in the patient's status treated appropriately?			
6. Was the dose & route of medication documented per policy?			
7. Was the MD notified of significant changes in patient's status?			
8. Was the MD response appropriate?			
9. Were all forms signed as required?			

FIGURE 6-2 | Conscious sedation quality improvement monitoring and evaluation. (Courtesy Holmes Medical Center.)

PRE-PROCEDURE

DATE: ___ TRANSFERRED: DATE_____ TIME_____ UNIT_____ BY_____ ARRIVAL: DATE_____ TIME_____ DEPT/UNIT_____ BY_____

Patient Statement of Procedure:

PSYCHOSOCIAL ASSESSMENT
ACCOMPANIED BY: ☐ Spouse ☐ Parent/Legal Guardian ☐ Law Enforcement Officer ☐ None
☐ Other _____

HT: ___ WT: ___ AGE: ___

COMMUNICATION LIMITATIONS:
☐ None ☐ Hearing _____ ☐ Visual _____
☐ Language Barrier, Speaks _____
☐ Other _____
Comments: _____

TEMP_____
☐ Oral
☐ Rectal
☐ Axillary
☐ Tympanic

PULSE _____
☐ Apical
☐ Radial

RESP _____

B/P _____

Allergies

Pregnancy Status ☐ Yes ☐ No ☐ NA

Consent Obtained ☐ Yes ☐ No

ID Bracelet Correct and Applied ☐ Yes ☐ No ☐ NA

Prosthetic Device: ☐ Yes ☐ No
If Yes, Type _____
Remove? ☐ Yes ☐ No
Last oral intake (food or fluid)
Date: _____
Time: _____

* PP   O-Absent   1-Thready   2-Normal   3-Full   4-Bounding

POSTERIOR TIBIAL   L___ R___
DORSALIS REDIS   L___ R___
POPLITEAL   L___ R___
BRACHIAL   L___ R___
FEMORAL   L___ R___

ASA Score: _____

Chief Complaint:

COMA SCALE

EYES OPEN	Spontaneously	
	To Speech	
	To Pain	
	None	
BEST VERBAL RESPONSE	Oriented	
	Confused	
	Inappropriate Words	
	Incomprehensible Snds	
	None	
BEST MOTOR RESPONSE	Obeys Commands	
	Localizes Pain	
	Flexion Withdrawal	
	Flexion	
	Extension	
	None	

REFLEXES

COMA SCORE

	RIGHT	SIZE
PUPILS		REACTION
	LEFT	SIZE
		REACTION
BABINSKI	RIGHT	
	LEFT	
CORNEAL	RIGHT	
	LEFT	
GAG		
COUGH		

PUPILS: 1 2 3 4 5 6 7 8
R = RIGHT
L = LEFT
B = BRISK
S = SLUGGISH
1 = PRESENT
# = ABSENT

LIMB MOVEMENT

ARMS
Normal Power
Mild Weakness
Severe Weakness
Spastic Flexion
Extension
No Response

LEGS
Normal Power
Mild Weakness
Severe Weakness
Spastic Flexion
Extension
No Response

Past Medical/Surgical History:

Past Anesthetics & Complications:

Skin: ☐ Warm ☐ Dry ☐ Moist ☐ Cold ☐ Pale ☐ Flushed ☐ Jaundiced ☐ Other _____

MEDICAL/NURSING INTERVENTIONS

LEGEND: 1-IV
2-NG TUBE
3-CHEST TUBE
4-FOLEY
5-A-LINE
6-CVP
7-SWAN-GANZ
8-WOUND DRAINS
9-WOUND DRAINS
A-ABRASIONS
B-BRUISES
C-LACERATIONS

FRONT   BACK

MEDICATIONS

TIME	DRUG	ROUTE	DOSE	RN/MD

IV ☐ Yes ☐ No ☐ NA   Solution
IV Started By:
Rate: Type/Gauge Needle:

PATIENT EDUCATION: ☐ Procedure: ☐ Medication

Patient ID

Harris County Hospital District
INTRAVENOUS CONSCIOUS/DEEP SEDATION
NURSING ASSESSMENT

280850 / HCHD-7139 (2/95)
Page 1

FIGURE 6-3 | Sample of IV conscious/deep sedation nursing assessment form. (Courtesy Harris County Hospital District.)   Continued

Harris County Hospital District
INTRA PROCEDURE

TIME	TREATMENTS/OBSERVATIONS		
		TIME	
		TEMP.	
		$\vee$ BP $\wedge$	220
		Pulse •	200
			180
		Resp. ○	160
		% 0 SAT •	140
			120
		EKG Leads	100
			80
			60
			40
			20
			16
			12
			8
			4
			0

Pathology: Specimen Sent to Lab:
☐ Yes ☐ No ☐ N/A

☐ Biopsy _____   ☐ Other(Specify)_____

☐ Polyp_____   ☐ Lavage_____   ☐ Brushing_____

RADIOLOGY						EQUIPMENT/ACCESSORIES: (with serial number)
PROCEDURE	CATHETER	CONTRAST	RATE/VOL/ACCEL	PROGRAM	CONTRAST COUNT	

INTAKE					OUTPUT		
TIME	SITE	SOLUTION	CC ADMIN	CC REMAINING	SOURCE	DESCRIPTION	DESCRIPTION

MEDICATION				
TIME	DRUG	DOSE	ROUTE	RN/MD

280850 / HCHD-7139 (2/95)
Page 2

FIGURE 6-3 cont'd | Sample of IV conscious/deep sedation nursing assessment form.

Harris County Hospital District
POST PROCEDURE

TIME	MEDICATIONS				ADMITTED
	DRUG	DOSE	ROUTE	NURSE	Date_____ Time _____ Unit _____ By _____

Anesthetic Agents _____

Time	LAB STUDIES

Allergies:

PAR SCORE

		IN	15	30	45	60	OUT

TIME

TEMP.

BP 220 / Pulse 200 / 180 / Resp. 160 / %0 SAT 140 / 120 / 100 / 80 / 60 / 40 / 20 / 16 / 12 / 8 / 4 / 0

MOTOR ACTIVITY
Active motion voluntarily on command — 2
Weak motion voluntarily on command — 1
No motion — 0

RESPIRATION
Coughing on command or crying — 2
Maintaining good airway — 1
Airway requires maintenance — 0

BLOOD PRESSURE
± 0-20MM HG of preanesthesic level — 2
± 20-50MM HG of preanesthesic level — 1
> 50MM HG of preanesthesic level — 0

CONSCIOUSNESS
Fully awake or easily arousable on calling — 2
Responding to stimuli and presence of protective reflexes — 1
Not responding or absence of protective reflexes — 0

COLOR
Pink — 2
Pale, dusky, blotchy — 1
Cyanotic — 0

TOTAL SCORE AT TIME OF TRANSFER/DISCHARGE FROM AREA OF RECOVERY _____
(PATIENT'S SCORE MUST BE ≥ 8 TO BE TRANSFERRED.)

IN ADDITION, PATIENTS DISCHARGE HOME MUST MEET THE FOLLOWING CRITERIA WITH A SCORE OF ≥8.

ACTIVITY
Ambulates independently or at preanesthetic activity level — 2
Ambulates with assistance or at preanesthetic activity level — 1
Cannot ambulate at preanesthetic level — 0

MENTAL STATUS
Oriented X 3 — 2
Oriented X 2 — 1
Oriented X 1 — 0

PAIN
Minimal (0-3 on a VAS numeric scale) — 2
Moderate (4-7 on a VAS numeric scale) — 1
Severe (7-10 on a VAS numeric scale)I — 0

NAUSEA / VOMITING
Absence of nausea and vomiting — 2
Presence of nausea without vomiting — 1
Presence of nausea and vomiting — 0

INTAKE / OUTPUT
Tolerates po fluids and voids — 2
Tolerates po fluids or voids — 1
Neither — 0

TOTAL SCORE PRIOR TO DISCHARGE _____ (MUST BE ≥ 16.)

INTAKE

TIME	SITE	SOLUTION	CC ADMIN	CC REMAINING	BASELINE Vital Signs:

OUTPUT

SOURCE	DESCRIPTION	TOTAL	DISCHARGED
			Date_____ Time_____ Unit_____
			DOCTOR:
			NURSE:

280850 / HCHD-7139 (2/95)
Page 3

FIGURE 6-3 cont'd | Sample of IV conscious/deep sedation nursing assessment form.

DUKE UNIVERSITY MEDICAL CENTER
CONSCIOUS SEDATION FLOW SHEET

Diagnosis: _____
Procedure: _____
Date: _____
Location: _____
Operator(s): _____

Addressograph

Page _____ of _____

PRE-PROCEDURE CHECKLIST AND BASELINE DATA
Check or fill in the value for each of the following as completed:

Informed consent for sedation signed _____
Current medication list reviewed _____
Relevant history and physical assessment documented _____
Pre-sedation assessment and plan documented _____
Post-sedation plan documented _____

Oxygen administered by	
None	_____
FM	_____
NP	_____

Prior Adverse Drug Reactions: _____ _____ _____
Premedications given: _____ _____ _____
NPO × _____ hours   Patient's Last Menstrual Period (date): _____   Weight: _____

Baseline LOC*: [_____]   *See Ramsey score on reverse side.
Baseline Vital Signs: Pulse: _____   R: _____   BP: _____ O_2Sat: _____%

PROCEDURE

Time Procedure Starts: [_____]   Time Procedure Ends: [_____]

Time	P	R	BP	O_2Sat	LOC	IV Fluids/Drugs/Doses/Route	Notes/Pt. Response	Signature

POST PROCEDURE

Time	P	R	BP	O_2Sat	LOC	IV Fluids/Drugs/Doses/Route	Notes/Pt. Response	Signature

Therapy Emergent Adverse Reactions/Management: _____

Discharge Instructions given to outpatient/family: YES [____]   Verbal Report given to/time: _____

Time of discharge/transfer: [_____]   **Signature/title of monitor:** _____

Ramsey score at discharge/transfer: [____]   **Signature and ID of M.D.:** _____

FIGURE 6-4 | Sample of conscious sedation flow sheet. (Courtesy Duke University Medical Center.)

Training and competency. This section should identify ongoing training and education requirements for health care providers responsible for managing the care of patients receiving conscious sedation and analgesia.

Appendices. This section should refer to any existing protocols as appropriate.

Bibliography. This section should identify any documents that have been used in the protocol revision.

Step 4: Communication

A request for multidisciplinary input of comments and suggestions on the draft version should be sent out to all departments before final administrative approval. Following the accepted process for administrative approval of the protocol, methods for informing and educating staff should be identified. All health care providers who may be affected by the revised standard of care should be informed and educated as appropriate. One of the most common forms of communication is the development of a required inservice educational program for all staff who are responsible for the management of patients receiving conscious sedation and analgesia.

Step 5: Outcome Evaluation

Part of the continuous quality improvement process should include a plan to monitor any variation from identified indicators and patient outcome. For example, if the standard of care did not recommend monitoring the patient, such an occurrence should be identified, and any effects on patient outcome and treatment should be documented and forwarded to appropriate channels for review (e.g., anesthesia committee).

Management of a patient receiving conscious sedation and analgesia is identified by the JCAHO as high-volume, high-risk, and problem-prone. A plan should be in place to measure and determine that the care delivered is attaining the desired patient effect. An institution should measure the outcome of patient care and identify the impact of the existing standard of care to determine if there are any opportunities for improvement.

CONCLUSION

An institution's standard of care during a procedure requiring the administration of conscious sedation and analgesia by a nonanesthesia provider should be written clearly and concisely (Box 6-1 and Figure 6-1). The care provided to the patient should be based on both national and local recommendations. The process for revising an existing standard of care is determined by the respective institution. However, the model suggested in Box 6-1 could be modified to facilitate revision of the standard of care. These standards of care work well and are intended for use at each respective institution. They can be used by other facilities as a benchmark for their

Text continued on p. 124

| BOX 6-1 | *Duke University Medical Center Policy on Conscious Sedation* |

A. INTENT

A policy with minimum requirements for administering and monitoring conscious sedation establishes "one standard of care" for all patients throughout the medical center. Site-specific conscious sedation guidelines may be more, *but not less,* restrictive than medical center guidelines, and must conform to requirements that patients with the same health status receive a comparable level of care throughout the medical center. These standards are not intended to address situations that require the services of a qualified, hospital credentialed anesthesia provider. This policy does not apply to care such as sedation in the intensive care unit (e.g., patients on ventilators), pain control, or when agents are given with the intent to provide anxiolysis only.

B. DEFINITIONS

1. *Conscious sedation* is produced by the administration of a drug or drugs which depress the level of consciousness (with or without providing analgesia) while retaining the ability to independently and continuously maintain a patent airway and to respond appropriately to verbal and physical stimuli. Adequate respiratory drive is maintained. Constant vigilance by the patient's monitor is required to avoid deeper levels of sedation and to assure safety of the patient undergoing a procedure requiring conscious sedation.
2. *Deep sedation* is a state of depressed consciousness from which the patient is not easily aroused and in which partial or complete loss of protective reflexes, including the ability to independently maintain a patent airway, may occur, and in which purposeful response to verbal or physical stimuli may not occur. Normal respiratory drive may be lost. *This level of sedation should NOT be the goal of conscious sedation, but undertaken only with the assistance of a qualified anesthesia provider.*

C. PROCEDURE EVALUATION

A medical history and physical examination must be performed and documented in the medical record. A plan for the operative or invasive procedure, presedation assessment, need for blood products, and postprocedure care needs must be documented in the chart.

D. PATIENT SELECTION

1. The need for any short-term therapeutic, diagnostic, or surgical procedure and subsequent use of conscious sedation will remain under the individual physician's (MD, DDS) practice direction.
2. There must be a documented preprocedure evaluation of the patient prior to any short-term therapeutic, diagnostic, or surgical procedure requiring conscious sedation.
3. Practitioners are encouraged to consult with a member of the Anesthesiology Department when there is a question regarding the appropriate delivery of conscious sedation.

Reprinted with permission of Duke University Medical Center, Durham, NC.

| BOX 6-1 | *Duke University Medical Center Policy on Conscious Sedation—cont'd* |

E. INFORMED CONSENT

1. The patient should be made aware of the risks associated with conscious sedation, analgesia, and anesthesia. The informed consent for any short-term therapeutic, diagnostic, or surgical procedure in which conscious sedation is to be employed should include the risks of conscious sedation, as appropriate. The consent form should be placed in the patient's chart as part of the permanent record. Consent for conscious sedation can be incorporated into any existing procedure-specific consent form, if the risks of sedation are specifically delineated.

F. MANAGEMENT

The care of patients receiving conscious sedation is based on these criteria below:

1. The practitioners responsible for the short-term therapeutic, diagnostic, or surgical procedure and/or the administration of drugs for conscious sedation shall be appropriately trained.
2. The Director of the care unit or service performing the procedure shall certify that all practitioners administering conscious sedation are trained in airway management and the safe use of drugs causing sedation.
3. The minimum number of available personnel for any procedure employing conscious sedation shall be two: the *operator* (person performing the procedure) and the *monitor* (an assistant trained to monitor appropriate physiological parameters and to assist in any supportive or resuscitative measures required). The monitor will not engage in any tasks that would compromise continuous patient monitoring. These personnel will be available to the patient from the time of administration of conscious sedation until recovery or the care of the patient is transferred to personnel performing recovery care.
4. The physician (MD, DDS) selects, orders, and signs the written order for the medication to produce conscious sedation.
5. The conscious sedation *monitor* must be able to monitor and respond appropriately to the patient's response to medication, including adverse drug reactions and, at a minimum, changes in:
   a. Vital signs
   b. Level of consciousness
   c. Presence or lack of a patent airway
   d. Oxygen saturation
   e. Patient's response to medication
6. A standardized conscious sedation flow sheet (chart) should be completed by the *monitor* for all patients receiving conscious sedation (see Figure 6-4).
7. Minimum monitoring shall include:
   - Blood pressure
   - Pulse and respiratory rates
   - Oxygen saturation (continuous monitoring with pulse oximetry)
   - Level of consciousness

Continued

BOX 6-1	*Duke University Medical Center Policy on Conscious Sedation—cont'd*

Baseline BP, pulse and respiratory rates, O_2 saturation (on room air unless the patient arrives with O_2), and level of consciousness must be documented on the flow sheet. BP, pulse and respiratory rates, O_2 saturation, and level of consciousness must be documented on the flow sheet at least every 10 minutes during the procedure and one minute following each additional dose of sedative medication given and more frequently as the patient's clinical needs dictate. Additional monitoring will be added at the physician's discretion.

8. The following minimum equipment must be present, in working order, and be ready for use in the room where conscious sedation is being administered.
   a. Oxygen
   b. Suction
   c. Emergency airway equipment
   d. Noninvasive BP monitor or manual BP cuff
   e. Pulse oximeter
   f. A cardiac arrest cart with defibrillator must be located in close proximity to the procedure/sedation site

9. All patients receiving intravenous conscious sedation must have a patent IV with continuous administration of IV fluids per physician's order. Patent "saline (or heparin) locks" are acceptable for patients with contraindications to IV fluids. IV fluid for resuscitation should be readily available. The need for IV access in patients receiving conscious sedation by any other route of administration shall be determined by the physician.

10. Documentation on the conscious sedation flow sheet must include:
   a. Informed consent signed
   b. Beginning and end time of procedure
   c. Name, dose, route, time of all drugs given
   d. Prior adverse drug reactions (including allergies)
   e. Premedication, time and effect
   f. All parameters given in section F
   g. Oxygen delivered; L/M via mask or nasal
   h. Any adverse drug reactions or untoward/significant responses. Management and outcome of these events. Patient response to all drugs given.

G. POSTPROCEDURE

1. Patients who receive conscious sedation should be monitored postprocedure. Patients will be *recovered* when specific criteria, indicating a return to safe physiological and psychological levels, have been achieved. Specifically, their vital signs, O_2 sat., and LOC are stable and within preprocedure limits OR their vital signs and O_2 sat. are stable and the Ramsey score is no higher than 3 (sedated but responsive to commands). The same flow sheet used during

conscious sedation should be continued throughout the postprocedure recovery phase. Recovery should be clearly documented prior to discharge. The ratio of patients to care givers in the postprocedure observation area should be appropriate to the patient's age, preprocedure condition, procedure performed, and amount of sedation administered.

  a. Inpatient monitoring and documentation requirements:

  (1) BP, HR, R, O_2 sat. (continuous monitoring) and level of consciousness at least every 15 minutes.

  (2) Vital signs, O_2 sat., level of consciousness that are stable and within preprocedure limits prior to return to ward.

  (3) Observe and document any postprocedure complications, management of those events, and patient response.

  (4) Document name, dose, time, and response of any drugs given in the postprocedure period.

  (5) Provide a verbal report to nurse caring for patient on return to patient care unit. Include preprocedure VS and LOC, any problems encountered during or postprocedure, total drugs given, IV fluid total, and status of IV. Note time and name of person to whom the report was given and sign flow sheet. Place in patient's permanent record.

  b. Outpatient monitoring and documentation requirements:

  (1) Same

  (2) Same, except applies to discharge

  (3) Same

  (4) Same

  (5) Provide verbal and written discharge instructions to patient and a responsible adult accompanying patient; have them verbalize understanding of the instructions. Document this on the flow sheet.

  (6) Document discharge VS, LOC, and status of IV on flow sheet; sign and place in patient's permanent medical record.

H. REVIEW/REVISION OF POLICY AND FORMS

This policy shall be reviewed and, if necessary, revised at least every three years.

  1. Policy review/revision shall be by the Anesthesiology Department and the Pharmacy and Therapeutics Committee with approval of the Executive Committee of the Medical Staff.

  2. Variances to the policy and flow sheets to meet the needs of specific departments may be allowed when the following conditions are met:

  a. All basic guidelines are maintained (e.g., individual department policies can be *more* but not *less* restrictive/specific).

  b. The variant policy or forms are approved by the Anesthesiology Department, the Pharmacy and Therapeutics Committee, and the Executive Committee of the Medical Center.

Continued

BOX 6-1 | *Duke University Medical Center Policy on Conscious Sedation—cont'd*

---

    c. All variant policies and forms are reviewed/revised and then approved by the above at least every three years.

3. Department specific versions of the consent form and patient discharge instructions are not allowed.

Approved by Director of Pharmacy

_____

Approved by Chairman, Anesthesiology Department

_____

Approved by Chief Operating Officer, Duke Hospital

_____

November 16, 1994.

---

standard of care for patients receiving conscious sedation and analgesia during a short-term diagnostic, therapeutic, or surgical procedure. The sample standards are not intended to be used as a replacement for any existing institution's standard of care for the patient receiving conscious sedation and analgesia.

REFERENCES

American Nurses Association (1991). *Position statement on the role of the registered nurse (RN) in the management of patients receiving IV conscious sedation for short-term therapeutic, diagnostic, or surgical procedures.* Washington, DC: Author.

Conscious sedation policy offers you a bench mark. (Oct., 1995). *Same-Day Surgery*, pp. 119-122.

Holland, C. A. (1995). Conscious sedation policy development and review. *Journal of the American Association of Nurse Anesthetists, 63*(3), 196-197.

Joint Commission on Accreditation of Healthcare Organizations (1996). *Comprehensive accreditation manual for hospitals.* Oakbrook Terrace, IL: Author.

Joint Commission on Accreditation of Healthcare Organizations (1994). Does sedation constitute anesthesia? Perspectives, *The Joint Commission Newsletter, 14*(3), pp. 10-11.

Competence in Patient Management

This chapter examines the concept of competence from the perspectives of education and nursing and as a requirement of the Joint Commission on the Accreditation of Healthcare Organizations (JCAHO). The JCAHO requires that health care organizations seeking accreditation have programs that assess, develop, and maintain competence. The chapter relates these perspectives to competencies for the registered nurse (RN) managing the care of a patient receiving intravenous (IV) conscious sedation and analgesia during a short-term therapeutic, diagnostic, or surgical procedure. The literature cited in this chapter supports the RN's role and associated practices. This chapter is not to be regarded as a source of common practices or as the sole legal, regulatory, accrediting, and/or credentialing reference on the subject. Readers who are establishing competencies and/or designing a competence-based activity in their organizations relative to this role should review local, state, and federal rules and regulations.

Competence is a contemporary issue. Education, nursing, and health care literature has consistently addressed competence in the last 15 years. These disciplines have taken different approaches to assessing, developing, and maintaining competence in practitioners, and each has designed activities and mechanisms to establish, facilitate, enhance, monitor, and measure competence in practitioners. Practitioners who are charged with designing competence-based activities or with developing competence in others should cross-reference the literature in all three fields to fully understand the concept of competence. It would be foolhardy, however, to think that competence could be developed by simply applying the activities suggested in the literature. Anyone who assumes there is a pragmatic, parochial quick-fix approach to competence will invariably accomplish the opposite of the intended goal—that is, incompetence. Competence is more than an attribute, a trait, a quality, or an ability. It is a process.

COMPETENCE IN EDUCATION

The value of competence-based education (CBE), like any other education discipline, lies in its service to society (Davis, 1992). In traditional education, a teacher plans, organizes, and conveys information to a student, who is tested on how much he or she has learned. The student (1) turns information into knowledge that is testable with a pen-and-pencil tool, (2) applies that knowledge to real-world situations (i.e., be able to perform), and (3) uses that knowledge to benefit society as a whole (i.e., problem-solve, make deliberate decisions, and think critically). If the student performs poorly on standardized tests or on the job, it is rare for a teacher in a traditional educational system to revise the planning, organization, and/or direction of information, even in an effort to improve outcomes.

Although CBE systems also plan, organize, and direct learning activities, in contrast to traditional educational programs, the learner's performance is used to evaluate the effectiveness of the activities. The philosophical basis of all CBE activities is to develop a learner's ability to *do* a job well (Davis, 1993). As such, *competency,* not competence, is at the core of CBE. Competency, as in the philosophy of CBE, is defined as integration of the knowledge, skills, and attitudes required for performance in a designated role and setting (Cyrs & Dobbert, 1976).

CBE and a variety of competence-based learning (CBL) models evolved during the 1960s as an approach to teacher education. It was believed that if students put what they were learning into real-world practice, they would be better able to successfully function in that position and in education as their life role. As early as 1973 educational research validated CBE as a philosophical approach to student teaching. Since then CBL models have also been implemented as outcome-based curricula for other fields, for example, performing arts, business, and nursing (e.g., Alverno College [Wisconsin] and Governor's State University [Illinois]). Research also identified some concepts inherent to all CBE systems and CBL models. One common concept is the teacher-as-manager of the learning environment. Three evolving concepts are individualized instruction, self-paced learning, and remediation. The learning environment is a rhetorical one in which the teacher uses task analysis, a learning needs assessment, and written objectives to plan activities and then chooses learning resources and teaching strategies to organize the information for the learner. This mirrors elements of traditional education: knowledge (educational design), skill (activity design and development), and performance-based criteria (teacher-as-facilitator and outcome evaluation).

As CBE and CBL models continue to be developed along educational lines, modifications in the original model and in the philosophy are likely to occur. Yet if persons who are charged with developing competence-based activities and/or are in charge of developing competence in others follow the founding principles of CBE, they will be successful and at the same time will help others to practice what they are learning while they are learning it.

COMPETENCE IN NURSING

The theme of safe patient care pervades all discussions of nursing—whether as an art or a science—regardless of an RN's basic educational preparation or continuing academic study, area of practice, or position or title. Safe patient care raises other questions related to life-long learning, continuing education, certification, and differentiated practice. Competence of the provider (i.e., the RN) and competence of the practice of nursing have only recently been addressed as issues in the literature. Formerly the term *competence* was always used to refer to behavioral models of CBE/CBL in which competenc*ies* were stated in measurable terms and students were involved in identifying learning resources and strategies.

In 1978 del Bueno compared the education principles of CBE/CBL with adult learning principles (Knowles, 1978). Based on her previous studies on competency in nursing cost-effectiveness (1975), on self-study as a method of inservice programs (1976), and on performance evaluations (1977), del Bueno concluded that CBL had two applications in validating the competency of an RN and competency in actual nursing practice. First, CBL can be used as a conceptual framework for a total curriculum; second, CBL can be used as a framework for a single learning unit/module. To date all the initial work by del Bueno has been used, refined, revised, and reported in the literature; more recently it has been designed as a computerized performance-based learning modality; most recently del Bueno has used her work to develop the critical thinking abilities of new graduates (1994).

In a separate but related investigation to identify a measurement-oriented approach to certify competence in nursing, Benner reported that "marked differences were found in the performance of beginning and experienced nurses. Beginning nurses viewed competency more simply—as the performance of basic skills that could be demonstrated in a laboratory setting. Experienced nurses, on the other hand, typically viewed competency in terms of performance in the actual practice settings" (Benner, 1982, p. 303). Noting the wide discrepancy between competence-based performance in the controlled settings students experienced versus competence-based performance in the real world of nursing practice, Benner developed the concepts of novice-to-expert and the RN's knowing-and-doing in nursing practice. Benner (1982) termed the competencies evident in actual clinical practice "abilities . . . that are identifiable as central to nursing" (p. 304) and was the first to suggest that these be "connected to specific patient outcomes" (p. 304). She addressed six limitations of CBE in relation to nursing and concluded that competencies cannot stand alone because they are not context-free talents or traits. Nonetheless, Benner's work, like del Bueno's, continues to be recognized in the competence literature as another method to assess competent providers and competent nursing practices.

In 1984 Alspach wrote an article relating CBE to the real world of nursing practice. The central characteristics of CBE, in relation to developing competence in human resources (i.e., RNs new to the critical care setting), are focused on "by redirecting the orientation process toward clinical rather than classroom performance" and are discussed in relation to the activity of orientation as a competence-based activity, that is, "a CBE approach to the critical care orientation process can improve program effectiveness and ultimately nursing care" (p. 657). Using a CBE approach to facilitate acquisition *and* application of knowledge, skills, and attitudes required for competence in critical care nursing modifies the traditional assessment, planning, implementation, evaluation steps of the education design process. Alspach promotes modification of these steps by integrating them with real-world standards, criteria, and performance. The four functional steps of education design with the CBE modifications as suggested by Alspach are listed in Table 7-1. In the classic article Alspach (1984) states, "Describing nursing interventions . . . and actually providing these interventions . . . are two very different examples of capability; the former can demonstrate knowledge, but only the latter can demonstrate competence" (p. 661).

Competence itself is required to manage the development of competence in others and to manage the design of competence programs. Health care systems are becoming health care businesses, and the business of health care mandates quality management systems and continuous performance improvement efforts. Competence of

TABLE 7-1 *Four Functional Steps of Education Design With Competency-Based Education Modifications*

FUNCTION	TRADITIONAL INTERPRETATION	CBE MODIFICATION
Assessment	What needs to be known in order to apply the information conveyed by the instructor	Examines what must be able to be done to perform the role in a safe, effective manner
Planning	In what sequence should the information be conveyed; what method of instruction should be used to convey the information	Includes the traditional content outline and consideration of the instruction; more important, it includes evaluation tools that preestablish performances to be demonstrated
Implementation	Presenting the information according to the plan toward achieving the assessed needs	Includes teaching and learning and adult education principles, with use of as many alternative and nontraditional types of learning tools as possible (i.e., self-directed modules)
Evaluation	Process and content tools	Uses the learner's performance against a set of criteria specified as standards for that performance, with emphasis on what is done (i.e., performance or the outcome* of what learners do with what learners know)

*Rodriguez and Stewart (1994) emphasize that "outcome" in relation to competence and nursing practice is not and should not be interpreted as outcome evaluation.

the organization and of its human resources (i.e., employees) is a priority as the future of health care as a business is managed and capitated. The literature must be appreciated as evolutionary; it must not be arbitrarily used by a novice level educator or beginning nursing staff developer.

Caution is advised in managing competence in others and in programs because the philosophical base of CBE is not the same as the conceptual use of CBE in the situational contexts of real-world nursing. It is different from modifying CBE as a competency-based approach to an educational activity such as orientation. The various definitions of the terms *competence, competency*, and *competencies* complicate the issue. Box 7-1 lists these terms and their common references in recent education and nursing literature.

COMPETENCE IN HEALTH CARE

The term *competent* first appeared in the JCAHO's *Accreditation Manual for Hospitals* in the early 1980s without any definition in its glossary. The term changed to *competence* in the 1986 manual and was defined in the glossary as "capacity according to requirement." Although this definition (but not its interpretation) changed slightly in the 1994 manual to "capacity equal to requirement," a fury of activity surrounded the 1986 publication. What was almost completely lost in the rush of articles and presentations on competence was the JCAHO's objective of organizational performance and the performance of its employees under its Agenda for Change initiative.

Before 1986 JCAHO accreditation status was based on structure standards. If an organization was able to demonstrate how the prescriptives of the JCAHO were met, the organization received accreditation. The most common way to demonstrate this

---

BOX 7-1 *Common Definitions*

Competence	A performance able to be demonstrated in a controlled or simulated situation (i.e., student laboratory, clinicals, and classroom didactic/practice sessions).
	—Capacity according to requirement (JCAHO, 1996)
Competency	Actual performance in a given work setting during the situational context of the work setting.
	—The knowledge, skills, and abilities necessary to fulfill the professional role functions of an RN in the perioperative setting (AORN, 1986)
Competencies	The individual performances that, when combined and as a whole, demonstrate competency.

JCAHO, Joint Commission on the Accreditation of Healthcare Organizations; *AORN,* Association of Operating Room Nurses.

was through a review of policies and procedures, which, by the mere fact of being in place and functional by a review of mortality and morbidity statistics, secured accreditation. Unfortunately, using such quantitative measures as morbidity and mortality statistics did not always demonstrate quality of care in a health care organization. Minimizing negative patient incidents such as falls, lengths of stay, and deaths did not support performance improvement activities toward positive patient outcomes within the organization. The JCAHO Agenda for Change was launched as a 10-year plan to change accreditation from a standards-based prescriptive process to an outcome-focused, quality-managed one. The goal of the Agenda for Change was twofold: (1) to decrease the competition between health care organizations to be all things to all people by increasing each organization's ability to do what it believes it does best and (2) to recognize that organizational performance as a whole is only as efficient and effective as the sum of its parts (i.e., the employees). According to performance improvement theory, if employees do their jobs, the organization is likewise able to do its job, that is, promote patient outcomes. The competence assessment programs for employees in all accredited health care organizations is important to organizational performance, which in turn is important to the accreditation process. The JCAHO standards for assessing competence are highlighted in Box 7-2. These standards, which are in the Human Resources section of the JCAHO manual, need to be supported by an interdisciplinary plan to meet the long-term effect of the performance-improvement initiative of the Agenda for Change. An orientation policy and procedure and a competence assessment policy and procedure need to be in place. Each should address how competence is (1) assessed, (2) developed, (3) maintained, and (4) documented in the organization and at unit level.

COMPETENCE IN MANAGING PATIENT CARE

A competence-based approach to managing the patient receiving IV conscious sedation and analgesia involves many variables, but not all of them can be addressed in this chapter. These variables include, but are not limited to, (1) the standards of practice that guide the RN, (2) the standards that guide the practice of anesthesia, (3)

BOX 7-2 *JCAHO Standards for Assessing Competence*

HR4	An orientation process provides initial job training and information and assesses the staff's ability to fulfill specified responsibilities.
HR4.2	Ongoing inservice and other education and training maintain and improve staff competence.
HR5	The hospital assesses each staff member's ability to meet performance expectations stated in his or her job description.

Data from Joint Commission on the Accreditation of Healthcare Organizations (1994). *Accreditation manual for hospitals.* Oakbrook Terrace, IL, p. 381.

the scope of practice of the RN, (4) the interdisciplinary process of mutual collaboration and communication between the nursing providers and the anesthesia providers within the organization, (5) the issue of competence in a given organization, and (6) mechanisms and systems within an organization that may and may not support an RN managing the care of the patient. However, for the purpose of discussion, it will be assumed that all variables have been explored and an ideal situation exists. This chapter addresses (1) the design of a competence-based educational activity for IV conscious sedation and analgesia that uses JCAHO criteria for programming, and (2) the development of an RN's competence to perform this role. Although either of these components can be used as action templates for novice-level clinical nurse educators and novice-level nursing staff developers, those who have already mastered the concepts of CBE, performance-as-competence in the situation context of nursing practice, and IV conscious sedation and analgesia as a knowledge/skill/ability equal to performance in the situational context of perioperative nursing can instead use this chapter to formulate action-research projects.

DESIGNING A COMPETENCE-BASED ACTIVITY

The design of a competence-based activity for IV conscious sedation and analgesia that meets or exceeds JCAHO criteria assumes that competence requires a knowledge base and a skill base and an understanding that the design of a competence-based activity requires considerations for caring and technical abilities. Competence in the caring and technical aspects of perioperative nursing practice is measured by the performance expectations of the job (Brazen, 1995); from the perspective of the JCAHO, competence is the ability to meet the requirements of the job. The template for a competence-based activity, complete with suggestions for the RN monitoring the patient receiving IV conscious sedation and analgesia, is shown in Fig. 7-1.

The global competence (i.e., *ability*) to "monitor a patient receiving intravenous conscious sedation" requires the ability to integrate one's knowledge competence with one's performance competence. A *knowledge-based competence* answers the question: What is the *thing* at the core of the job to be done? (i.e., what the RN needs to learn to *do*). The information an RN needs to know to monitor the patient safely and effectively can be stated as, "principles and practices of monitoring a patient receiving IV conscious sedation and analgesia."

At this point it seems prudent to acknowledge that the preceding statements regarding monitoring a patient receiving conscious sedation and analgesia may seem too simple. The reader is cautioned to remember that the example given in Figure 7-1 was created and developed by professionals well versed in CBE principles, practices, and theory; adult education principles, practices, and theory; and mastery-level perioperative nursing.

Since the underlying principle of any competence-based activity is the learner's accountability and responsibility for the information, it is not unusual for a knowl-

COMPETENCE: MONITORING THE PATIENT RECEIVING IVCS

KNOWLEDGE COMPETENCE

Principals and practices of monitoring

a patient receiving IVCS

LEARNING RESOURCES

(1) Organization/unit policy/procedure

(2) AORN recommended practices:

    (a) Managing the patient receiving intravenous conscious sedation/analgesia

    (b) Monitoring the patient receiving local anesthesia

(3) AORN standards:

    (a) Patient outcome standards

    (b) Clinical practice standards

(4) Independent study module

(5) Professional journals

PERFORMANCE COMPETENCIES

_____ Collects patient health data

_____ Identifies expected outcomes

_____ Develops a plan of care

_____ Implements the care

_____ Evaluates nursing intervention

_____ Describes the goals and objectives of IVCS

_____ Notes response(s) to IVCS

    _____ Physiologic

    _____ Psychologic

_____ Notes responses to drugs

_____ Provides anticipatory guidance for situational changes

_____ Uses resuscitation equipment

_____ Uses monitoring equipment

_____ Documents IVCS patient care

VALIDATION

Complete a knowledge test with a minimum of a 90% score.*

Complete an observation of performance competencies at a 100% score.*

(*) Remediation available ×1; alternate testing after one remediation

PARTICIPANT SIGNATURE _____

VALIDATOR SIGNATURE _____

DATE _____

FIGURE 7-1 | Template for competency-based activity.

edge competence to be stated in such general terms as "principles and practices." The competence-based activity for monitoring IV sedation and analgesia uses these general terms because the participant (the RN) in this activity is established and (theoretically) has already achieved competence in the psychosocial and humanistic sciences. An option for designing a competence-based activity to meet the knowledge needs would be to take a technical/task-oriented approach (e.g., "monitor the patient's physiological status"). If this is needed, as it may be in facilities with short-stay or same-day units, then any and all knowledge-competences for the RNs in these facilities would follow the same format (i.e., systems) and the performance-competencies would reflect the technical/task-oriented nature of the job. Given the current changes in health care and the ongoing discussion about licensed versus unlicensed providers, perioperative and critical care RNs may be philosophically uneasy with the technical/task-oriented approach. However, it may be the way for some facilities to keep the RN position secure because only an RN is able to assess the patient's outcome within a technical/task-oriented practice setting.

The *skill-based competence,* also referred to as the performance competence, answers the question: What is critical *to do* to show how the core of the job (i.e., essential information) is accomplished effectively and safely? If a competence-based activity is designed as an initial educational experience in developing competence (e.g., orientation or because of a change in role or responsibility), the performance competencies need to involve a step-by-step approach. Itemized instructions would include basic checks such as whether the monitoring device is plugged in and the placement of each lead and cuff is done correctly. If, on the other hand, the activity is designed as an ongoing competence assessment or a maintenance tool, the list of performance competencies may take a more general approach. Effectiveness of performance (rather than safety) is the focus that determines if competence is being assessed or if maintenance of competence is the primary goal of the activity. Germane to performance competencies is that once the performer gains expertise, the performer chooses which of many possible actions is actually needed to be performed. Designing activities to assess competence and/or maintain competence (and thereby determine the effectiveness of the performance) in the expert-level perioperative RN is much less formidable than designing activities to develop competence (and in so doing determine if the participant is providing a "safe" level of care).

The *learning resources* of a competence-based activity include all the resources and references the learner can access to prepare for validation of the competence. The designer of an activity should include only those resources and references that (1) address the facility/unit performance expectations and (2) will be used to create the written test. Including every resource and reference would overwhelm even an expert adult learner. Adults who are learners in competence-based activities are accountable and responsible for seeking information they specifically need to succeed. Therefore the educator must act as a facilitator and as such may directly obtain requested information, arrange a learning experience to meet the learner's request, or individualize the activity to meet the expressed needs of the learner. Additional resources and references should be listed on the design of the activity because in some facilities and units monitoring the patient receiving IV conscious sedation and analgesia is a full-time performance. Although the ever-expanding practice of an RN in such a care setting would increase expertise as well as competence, it is also likely that the RN would need advanced knowledge-based competence in monitoring the patient.

Competence *validation* is accomplished through a combination of paper-and-pencil testing and observation of performance, with validation not necessarily occurring simultaneously. Although the percentile score necessary to validate competence is arbitrary, it should be in direct proportion to the risk(s) associated with the practice. For example, in some practice settings where it is rare for an RN to monitor a patient receiving IV conscious sedation and analgesia, the RN may monitor only patients who are classified by an anesthesia provider as "healthy with no other existing illness." In this setting the RNs, who have no other responsibilities during the surgical intervention/invasive procedure than to monitor the patient according to unit-specific policy, procedure, and protocol, may need to achieve a different score than RNs in another facility, who are monitoring at-risk patients. Knowledge-based competence must be viewed in relation to the perceived risks associated with the specific client base (e.g., predominantly healthy? having multiple medical diseases? predominantly requiring a certain type of surgical intervention or invasive procedure? requiring support systems predischarge and postdischarge?).

Although paper-and-pencil testing is not the only way to validate knowledge-based competence, it is the most commonly used tool. One obvious advantage is that once the initial time is invested in creating and testing the tool, it becomes an economical, low-maintenance standardized item that is specific to the facility or unit and practice. The disadvantage is that paper-and-pencil testing is not perceived as being as stimulating as, for example, an interactive computer-based activity. Over time, as electronic testing becomes less expensive, the linear-thinking approach may change. Until then multiple-choice and fill-in-the-blank testing to validate knowledge competence will continue to be done with paper and pencil.

Likewise, performance competencies are categorized as inclusive or exclusive, depending on whether the focus of the competence-based activity is (1) the safety of the patient population as a whole or (2) the effectiveness of the care given to the population of patients served. If the competence of the RN to monitor the patient safely is of primary concern, the performance competencies to be demonstrated and observed need to be highly detailed. If the competence of the RN to give care effectively is of primary concern, performance competencies to be demonstrated and observed can be stated in general terms. Since the competence of the RN whose only responsibility is to monitor the patient receiving IV conscious sedation and analgesia is a multidimensional issue, much like that of competence, it is not unusual to have two separate competence-based activities. When a novice-level clinical RN is being oriented to the role of monitoring such a patient, safety is the focus of the competence. Therefore the RN would need to achieve validation of his or her knowledge and performance to safely monitor healthy, short-stay patients. However, as this same novice-level clinician gains expertise, he or she will achieve competence validation in "effectively" monitoring patients with multiple and/or diverse care needs. Since in most situations competence in both safe care and effective care needs to be achieved, a time frame for each could be established that would be as facility specific or unit specific as necessary.

The issue of who should be validating whom with regard to the competence of monitoring a patient receiving IV conscious sedation and analgesia needs to be resolved through interdisciplinary discussions between the nursing care providers and the anesthesia care providers at facilities or in units where this is an issue. Currently, the nursing literature supports nurses validating nursing practice. If RNs do not validate nursing care, how will RNs be able to associate performance competencies with patient outcomes?

The final design of any competence-based activity can be evaluated with the tool outlined in Figure 7-2, but the design should also be subjected to a pilot test in the actual work setting. It is strongly suggested that (1) the design be explained with the term *competence* as it is used in CBE and by JCAHO, (2) a consensus (not majority opinion) be reached on the performance competencies, and (3) a summary document addressing the need for the activity and its format be created and used as a performance-improvement program.

DEVELOPING RN COMPETENCE TO MONITOR PATIENTS

It has been asserted by del Bueno (1994) that regardless of the type of nursing program, it is not reasonable to expect new graduates to be competent; however, it is reasonable to expect them to be able to (1) identify essential clinical data indicative of acute changes in patient health status, (2) initiate independent and collaborative actions to correct or minimize any risks to the patient's health, (3) know why the actions are relevant, and (4) differentiate patient problems needing immediate or subsequent action. In the continuum of nursing practice, the Association of Operating Room Nurses (AORN) Advanced Practice Competencies (1996a) include:

> (1) managing comprehensive and individualized care through the perioperative continuum by using [both] in-depth knowledge from the natural and behavioral sciences with clinical experience as the foundation for perioperative care, (2) using selected interpersonal theories and strategies to promote positive client interactions and outcomes by establishing a healing environment, and (3) demonstrating knowledge of (a) learning theories, (b) human behavior, (c) change theory, (d) stress and coping mechanisms, (e) crises management, (f) human family development and interactions, and (g) health issues (pp. 88-90)

Developing RN competence to monitor a patient receiving IV conscious sedation and analgesia must begin with an assessment of the RN's experience in relation to

EVALUATION TOOL FOR COMPETENCY-BASED ACTIVITY

_____At a minimum, were at least two of the following used to create this competence-based activity?

    _____Standards of Practice

    _____National Guideline

    _____National Position Statement

    _____National Recommended Practices

    _____Job Descriptions

    _____Regulatory/accrediting Agency Criteria

    _____Formal Learning Needs Assessment

    _____Quality Management Indicators

_____Does the competence statement reflect an ability a person can-do-a-what-they're-supposed-to-do and when-they're-supposed-to-do-it?

_____ Does the knowledge-based competence statement capture essential need-to-know information?

_____Are each of the performance competencies able to be demonstrated and observed, ie, measurable?

_____Are at least two of the following available to validate competence?

    _____Written tests

    _____Preceptors

    _____Checklists

    _____Demonstration and return

    _____Peer Review

_____Is the opportunity for remediation acknowledged?

_____Are the learning resources accessible to participants?

_____Are the learning resources for remediation accessible to participants?

_____Are the learning resources/references for alternate testing available?

_____Have all of the following been achieved:

    _____Consensus opinion

    _____Pilot-testing

    _____Summative Description

FIGURE 7-2 | Evaluation tool for competency-based activity.

the competence(s) required of the job, which, in turn, will make obvious his or her learning needs. Once the learning needs are identified, activities specifically designed to meet those needs can be planned, implemented, and evaluated using a competence-based activity. An RN who is new to the professional role will likely need two types of assessment, one to the expectations of the role and one to the responsibilities of the role. This person will need more guided learning experiences to achieve the competence than will an experienced RN. These experiences may be best supported by encouraging the RN to self-study IV conscious sedation and analgesia in addition to having him or her work with a preceptor or with an RN anesthetist. The experienced RN should be encouraged to transfer as much information as possible and to use self-directed learning methods.

The RN who is new to the role of monitoring patients receiving IV conscious sedation and analgesia may feel overwhelmed and may attempt to meet too many of the patient's psychosocial needs in lieu of his or her clinical needs or vice versa. The RN should not be put in such a compromising situation until he or she has had the opportunity to gain experience in more routine clinical perioperative nursing. On the other hand, it should never be assumed that an RN is able to function as the monitoring RN simply on the basis of overall experience. It is well known that the safety of a patient should never be compromised because of staffing, yet rarely is this issue addressed in policy, procedure, or protocol. It is still too often the case that an RN must simultaneously monitor and circulate, or an RN whose competence has not been validated is assigned to monitor. Even if a facility or unit is unable to afford the luxury of an educator or staff development RN, it is still an expectation of a professional to engage in ongoing learning and to share what is learned with peers and colleagues (AORN, 1996b). If monitoring a patient receiving IV conscious sedation and analgesia is not a competence in a work setting but monitoring such a patient is an expectation, the resources and references listed in Fig. 7-1 can be used for self-study.

In summary, developing an RN's competence to monitor patients receiving IV conscious sedation and analgesia is no different from developing competence to practice nursing. This chapter is a guide for the minimal knowledge and performance that must be demonstrated to achieve competence. The resources and references given in Figure 7-1 and the examples of other competence designs in the Bibliography of this chapter, even though not specific to a work setting, all can be used as catalysts for change.

CONCLUSION

During IV conscious sedation and analgesia, a patient should be able to respond to verbal or physical commands and to maintain a patent airway. Because of patient variation in illness, age, and/or drug sensitivity, such patient responses may vary. Thus, IV conscious sedation and analgesia also must encompass continuous monitoring and intervention to safeguard the patient and to maintain positive patient outcomes (Cunningham, 1996). The use of an RN to monitor a patient receiving IV conscious sedation and analgesia is acceptable in most work settings, but the competence of the RN to do so is an issue that deserves to be considered. The actions of the RN, who is usually an employee of the hospital, must be within policies and procedures; the JCAHO requires hospitals to have an orientation and competence assessment policy and procedure in place. Neither the JCAHO requirement nor the practice of an RN as a monitoring nurse is new, but very little formal action has occurred in work settings to address the issue. At minimum, this chapter has raised an awareness of the concepts of competence and some basic approaches to be used in any work setting. At most, this chapter is an additional reference for those charged with developing competence-based activities or developing competence in others.

REFERENCES

Alspach, J. (1984). Designing a competency-based orientation for critical care nurses. *Heart and Lung, 13*(6), 655-662.

Association of Operating Room Nurses (1996a). Perioperative advanced practice nurse competency statements. In *AORN standards and recommended practices,* Denver, CO: Author.

Association of Operating Room Nurses (1996b). Standards of perioperative professional performance. In *AORN standards and recommended practices,* Denver, CO: Author.

Benner, P. (1982). Issues in competency-based testing. *Nursing Outlook, 30*(5),305-309.

Brazen, L. (1995). *Competence: It's not an option anymore!* AORN continuing education seminar. Corpus Christi, TX.

Cunningham, M.C. (1996). Conscious sedation AKA procedural sedation. In *The manual on anesthesia services,* Hot Springs National Park, AR: St. Joseph Regional Health Center.

Cyrs, T.E., & Dobbert, D.J. (1976). *A competency-based curriculum: What is it?* College of Pharmacy dissertation, University of Minnesota, Minneapolis.

Davis, J. (1993). Classroom discussion: Outcomes assessment. University of Denver, Denver, CO.

Davis, J. (1992). Classroom discussion: Curriculum. University of Denver, Denver, CO.

del Bueno, D. (1994). Why can't new grads think like nurses? *Nurse Educator, 19*(4), 9.

del Bueno, D. (1977). Performance evaluation: When all is said and done, more is said than done. *Journal of Nursing Administration, 7,* 21-23.

del Bueno, D. (1976). No more Wednesday matinees. *Nursing Outlook, 24,* 359-361.

del Bueno, D. (1975). The cost of competency. *Journal of Nursing Administration, 5,* 16-17.

del Bueno, D., Baker, R.F., & Christomyer, C. (1980). Implementing a competency-based orientation program. *Nurse Educator, 11*(5), 16-20.

Joint Commission on Accreditation of Healthcare Organizations (1983, 1986, 1994). *Accreditation manual for hospitals.* Oakbrook Terrace, IL: Author.

Knowles, M. (1978). *The modern practice of adult education: From pedagogy to androgyny.* Chicago: Associated Press/Follette Publishing Co.

Rodriguez, L., & Stewart, P. (1994). *Competency: What is it and how will I know it when I see it?* Eighth Annual Convention on Staff Development, Mosby Division of Continuing Education and Training, Las Vegas, NV.

BIBLIOGRAPHY

Calinno, C., Clifford, D. W., & Titano, K. (1995). Oxygen therapy giving you patient breathing room. *Nursing 95, 25*(12), 33-38.

Comer, D. M. (1992). Pulse oximetry: Implications for practice. *Journal of Obstetric, Gynecologic, & Neonatal Nursing, 21*(1), 35-41.

Ford, L. A., Wickham, V. A., & Clover, C. (1992). Developing a skills fair workshop: Enhancing competency performance. *Dimensions of Critical Care Nursing, 11*(6), 340-346.

Grauer, K., & Cavallaro, D. (1993). Intravenous access. In K. Grauer, & D. Cavallaro, *ACLS certification preparation* (3rd ed., Vol. 1). St. Louis: Mosby Lifeline.

Grauer, K., & Cavallaro, D. (1993). Management of airway and ventilation. In K. Grauer & D. Cavallaro, *ACLS certification preparation* (3rd ed., Vol. 1). St. Louis: Mosby Lifeline.

Miracle, V. A., & Allnutt, D. R. (1990). How to perform basic airway management. *Nursing 90, 20*(4), 55-60.

Saver, C. L., & Hurray, J. M. (1990). Electrocardiogram monitoring: Interpreting abnormal cardiac rhythms. *AORN Journal, 52*(2), 273-283.

Sims, J. (1996). Making sense of pulse oximetry and oxygen dissociation curve. *Nursing Times, 92*(1), 34-35.

Weinberg, L. A., & Stone-Griffith, S. Alternate methods of teaching: Use of self-learning packets. *Journal of Post Anesthesia Nursing, 7*(6), 392-397.

Witman, M. (1995). The push is on delivering medications safely by I.V. bolus. *Nursing 95, 25*(8), 52-54.

Pediatric Sedation

The patient under conscious sedation and analgesia "exhibits a depressed level of consciousness, but retains the ability to independently and continuously maintain a patent airway and respond appropriately to verbal commands or physical stimulation" (American Nurses Association, 1991). In the past patient selection for nurse-monitored sedation generally included clinical conditions that allowed for a wide safety margin and predictability. Patients were healthy, over the age of 18, and without compromising systemic problems. Today registered nurses (RNs) and other nonanesthesia providers are monitoring acutely ill patients and those younger than 18 years. Proper education and training and the following of appropriate guidelines allow the nonanesthesia provider and physician to collaborate in the delivery of a safe sedation level for the pediatric patient undergoing diagnostic, therapeutic, or minor surgical procedures.

The pediatric population presents many challenges for the nonanesthesia provider responsible for monitoring and administering medications. Even though providers may have little or no experience and expertise with pediatric patients, they often must administer medications for which pharmaceutical companies provide little dosage information. Therefore providers must be knowledgeable about how the pediatric population differs from adult patients anatomically and physiologically.

If anesthesia personnel are unavailable to manage the care of the pediatric patient scheduled for conscious sedation and analgesia, the next most appropriate provider is the RN. The RN should have a clear understanding of patient outcomes and the desirable effects of conscious sedation and analgesia. These effects include alteration in perception of pain, maintenance of intact protective reflexes, initiation of slurred speech, easy arousal from sleep, and minor variations in vital signs. Certain procedures call for a more deeply sedated patient. Because the risks of deep sedation are similar to those of general anesthesia, the patient should be monitored by professionals trained in pediatric basic life support and having proficient skills to manage a pediatric airway (U.S. Department of Health and Human Services, 1992, p. 46). Deep sedation is "a medically controlled state of depressed consciousness or unconsciousness from which the patient is not easily aroused. It may be accompanied by a partial or complete loss of protective reflexes, and includes the inability to maintain a patent airway independently and respond purposefully to physical stimulation or verbal command" (American Academy of Pediatrics, 1992).

A fine line exists between conscious sedation and deep sedation, and continuous uninterrupted monitoring by the RN is imperative. Continuous assessment should include observation, monitoring, and administering medications and documenting their effects on the patient. Minimal monitoring parameters include respiratory rate, oxygen saturation, blood pressure, cardiac rate and rhythm, level of consciousness, and skin condition (Association of Operating Room Nurses, 1997). Documentation should occur at 5- to 15-minute intervals and should include monitoring parameters, medications administered, time, route, and level of consciousness (e.g., crying, awake and peaceful, drowsy, sleeping but arousable).

GUIDELINES

The following guidelines incorporate recommendations from the American Academy of Pediatrics (1992) and the guidelines endorsed by 23 specialty nursing organizations (see Chapter 1). These recommendations provide for an optimal achievable level of care for the RN monitoring the pediatric patient. The types of procedures vary and may be performed with or without local anesthesia in a variety of settings (e.g., emergency department, operating surgical suite, medical-surgical unit, catheterization laboratory, pediatric unit, endoscopy laboratory, critical care unit). Medications should be administered under the direction and in the presence of a physician. Serious complications may arise at any time during the administration of medications for conscious sedation and analgesia. Therefore care is directed toward the prevention of these complications, which include (but are not limited to) hypoventilation, apnea, respiratory arrest, hypotension, allergic reaction, and cardiac depression.

Goals

The RN should be familiar with the goals of sedation for the pediatric patient, which are similar to those for the adult patient. These include (American Academy of Pediatrics, 1992) the following:

Ensure patient safety and welfare. Safe sedation of the pediatric patient is of primary concern. Consideration must be given to patient selection, skilled nursing staff, appropriate monitoring equipment, selective administration of medications, and preparedness to intervene in the event of an untoward effect.

Minimize physical discomfort or pain. Most pediatric patients who understand pain will ask, "Will it hurt?" How the RN manages the child's pain will influence the child's reaction to future procedures. During a painful procedure opioids are frequently administered to alter the pain threshold by providing analgesia during and following the procedure.

Minimize negative psychologic responses. The patient should be provided with proper analgesia and emotional support throughout the perioperative period to decrease the negative psychologic responses.

Maximize potential for amnesia. Many medications are selected for their amnesic effects. Benzodiazepines are frequently administered for the excellent anxiolysis and amnesic effects they provide to the patient.

Control behavior. Administration of selective medications can often control pain and thus behavior, lessening the need for physical restraint.

Discharge safely. The patient receiving conscious sedation and analgesia should be monitored for an appropriate period of time. Recommended discharge criteria should be determined and met before the child is allowed to return to the unit or home. The American Academy of Pediatrics (1992, p. 1114) recommends the following criteria for discharge:

1. Cardiovascular function and airway patency are satisfactory and stable.
2. The patient is easily arousable, and protective reflexes are intact.
3. The patient can talk (if age-appropriate).
4. The patient can sit up unaided (if age-appropriate).
5. For a very young or disabled child, incapable of the usual expected responses, the presedation level of responsiveness or a level as close as possible to the normal level for that child should be achieved.
6. The state of hydration is adequate.

Patient Selection

Appropriate patient selection is critical. Requiring staff to monitor a patient who is beyond their skill and knowledge level places the patient, RN, physician, and institution at legal risk. Patient selection criteria or categories may be part of an institution's policy and procedure on conscious sedation and analgesia. Patient selection for RN-monitored pediatric sedation and analgesia should include patients who are healthy or have only mild systemic disease. The classification system of patient physical status by the American Society of Anesthesiologists (ASA) is commonly used to determine appropriate patient categories for RN-monitored sedation (see Chapter 2). A normal healthy patient and a patient with mild systemic disease that is medically controlled and presents no contraindications for conscious sedation and analgesia or for the procedure to be performed are appropriate candidates for nurse-monitored sedation. Patients with severe systemic disease should be assessed individually to determine the appropriateness of RN-monitored sedation.

Personnel and Facility

Both the physician and the RN managing the care of the patient should be trained and adequately prepared to deal with life-threatening emergency situations (Yaster et al., 1990). A minimum of three persons should attend the pediatric patient, including a monitoring RN or anesthesia provider, who provides continuous uninterrupted monitoring of physiologic parameters throughout the procedure; an additional provider to assist during the procedure as necessary; and the physician performing the therapeutic, surgical, or diagnostic procedure. The physician performing the procedure should not be expected to also monitor the patient because most procedures require the physician's undivided attention. Depending on the type of procedure, a fourth person, such as an RN first assistant or physician assistant, may be required to assist.

The physician should be skilled in the appropriate selection of pediatric medications and trained in the management of complications related to conscious sedation and analgesia. Training should include pediatric basic life support and (ideally) pediatric advanced life support, which includes skills for the management of a pediatric airway, use of positive-pressure ventilation, insertion of oropharyngeal and nasopharyngeal airways, and endotracheal intubation (Holzman et al., 1994, p. 266).

To minimize risks to the patient, the monitoring RN should be knowledgeable about all medications that might be administered to the pediatric patient. These medications include single doses or combinations of sedatives, hypnotics, tranquilizers, and opioids. The RN should be familiar with each medication—understand the indications, contraindications, adverse reactions and their management, drug interactions, and acceptable pediatric dose range. The RN providing care for the pediatric patient should be competent in the following areas:

Pediatric basic life support (cardiopulmonary resuscitation)

Airway management

Patient assessment

Recognition of potential complications

Cardiac dysrhythmia interpretation

Pediatric advanced cardiac life support (recommended)

Emergency medications and emergency equipment to treat life-threatening complications should be immediately available. Essential equipment that should be present in the room includes a positive-pressure oxygen delivery system capable of delivering 90% oxygen or greater for a period of at least 60 minutes and an appropriate source of suction. Reversal medications should also be immediately available in the room. If the facility is free standing, written protocols should include patient transportation to an acute care facility (e.g., ambulance).

PREPROCEDURE ASSESSMENT

The pediatric patient should be assessed by the monitoring RN before the administration of conscious sedation and analgesia medications. The main purpose of the preprocedure assessment is to evaluate the patient to determine any known or unknown risk factors and to determine the appropriateness of RN monitoring for the patient. The following baseline health data are to be completed or obtained by the monitoring RN: (1) physical assessment, (2) current medications, (3) known drug allergies, (4) current medical condition, (5) past hospitalizations, (6) relevant family history, (7) fasting status, (8) communication level, (9) pain assessment, (10) signed informed consent, (11) pediatrician or family physician and telephone number, and (12) preparedness of child for the procedure.

The monitoring RN should be familiar with the patient's history and physical examination, height and weight, and baseline vital signs (i.e., respiratory rate, heart rate and rhythm, oxygen saturation, blood pressure, level of consciousness, and skin condition). Additional assessment of the airway should include asking a child who is able to sit upright to look at the ceiling to determine if the child has any difficulty hyperextending the neck or has decreased neck or jaw mobility. The RN should also ask the child to open the mouth widely to assess for difficulty in opening the mouth and for loose teeth. Assessing the airway may be difficult with the very young patient. Any abnormal anatomic findings should be documented and reported to the physician.

The patient's fasting history is important and should be emphasized when gathering the information from both the child and the parent or responsible person. Fasting guidelines include clear liquids up to 3 hours before the procedure (Table 8-1). The patient is at risk for aspiration of gastric contents if an appropriate period of time for gastric emptying has not occurred.

In an emergency situation the physician must determine whether the risks of delaying the procedure outweigh the potential risks for aspiration. Although light sedation and local anesthetic may be used, there are other risk factors that may increase the chance of aspiration. These risks include "obesity, gastrointestinal obstruction, prior esophageal surgery, trauma, (particularly head trauma), neurologic dysfunction, and the administration of narcotics or sedatives which may decrease gastric motility or produce loss of consciousness or protective airway reflexes" (Coté, 1990, p. 47). Because of these risk factors, the emergent situation, and the possibility of en-

TABLE 8-1 *Fasting Guidelines*

AGE	MILK/SOLIDS	CLEAR LIQUIDS
<6 mo	4 hr	2 hr
6-36 mo	6 hr	3 hr
>36 mo	8 hr	3 hr

From Coté, C. J. (1994). Sedation for the pediatric patient: A review. *Pediatric Clinics of North America, 41*(1), 46.
NOTE: Most children older than 6 months can fast from milk and solids after midnight. Any amount of clear liquids (apple juice, water, sugar water) should be offered up to 3 hours before the scheduled procedure. If the procedure is scheduled for 10 AM, clear liquids should be given up to 7 AM.

dotracheal intubation, the most appropriate monitoring of the pediatric patient not meeting fasting guidelines should be provided by an anesthesia provider.

INTRAPROCEDURE ASSESSMENT

More than 23 nursing specialty organizations support the Position Statement on the Role of the Registered Nurse (RN) in the Management of Patients Receiving IV Conscious Sedation for Short-Term Therapeutic, Diagnostic, or Surgical Procedures, which states: "The nurse managing the care of the patient should have no other responsibilities that would leave the patient unattended or compromise continuous monitoring" (American Nurses Association, 1991). Therefore one nurse responsible for monitoring the patient should be provided throughout the procedure. The following monitoring parameters should be obtained and documented throughout the procedure: oxygen saturation, heart rate and rhythm, respiratory rate, blood pressure, level of consciousness, and skin color.

Because medications administered for conscious sedation and analgesia may result in decreased respirations or respiratory distress, close, continuous visual mon-

---

TABLE 8-2 *Signs and Symptoms of Respiratory Distress in the Pediatric Patient*

	MILD RESPIRATORY DISTRESS	MODERATE RESPIRATORY DISTRESS	SEVERE RESPIRATORY DISTRESS	RESPIRATORY FAILURE
Appearance/level of consciousness	Alert	Alert or may be confused	Lethargic	Unresponsive
Skin color and color of mucous membranes	Pink	Pink or cyanotic	Cyanotic	Cyanotic
Respiratory rate	Mildly increased	Mildly to moderately increased	Markedly increased	Decreased or apneic
Work of breathing	Subcostal retractions	Subcostal retractions Intercostal and sternal retractions Nasal flaring	Subcostal retractions Intercostal and sternal retractions Nasal flaring Suprasternal retractions	Decreased respiratory effort or none
Heart rate	Mildly increased	Mild to moderately increased	Markedly increased	Decreased

From Grauer, K., & Cavallaro, D. (1993). *ACLS: A comprehensive review* (3rd ed., Vol. 2, p. 626). St. Louis: Mosby.

itoring is critical. The monitoring RN should conduct frequent periodic assessments to ensure airway patency. Care should be taken that restraining devices, drapes, and equipment do not block the ability of the RN to visually assess the patient's respiratory and ventilatory status. Table 8-2 identifies five assessment parameters to aid in determining respiratory distress in the pediatric patient. Although the pulse oximeter is used as an aid in providing early warning of hypoxemia, the RN should also closely monitor skin color and the color of mucous membrane.

POSTPROCEDURE ASSESSMENT

The patient should be safely transported to the designated recovery area until the criteria for discharge are met. The same monitoring parameters previously described should be obtained until the patient is alert and responsive (i.e., oxygen saturation, heart rate and rhythm, respiratory rate, blood pressure, level of consciousness, and skin color). Before the patient is discharged, written discharge instructions should be provided to the parent or responsible escort.

MEDICATION ADMINISTRATION

Selection of medications and route of administration are determined by the physician. Many medications administered for conscious sedation and analgesia are not approved for pediatric use as evidenced by the information presented in the *Physicians' Desk Reference (PDR)* and the pharmaceutical package insert material. Detailed research involving appropriate clinical trials is required by the Food and Drug Administration before recommended dosages may appear in the *PDR* and pharmaceutical educational materials. However, this does not prevent the administration of such medications to populations for which little research exists. The physician is responsible for the selection of such medications, and the monitoring RN should be trained and familiar with each medication.

Determination of Dosage

The physician is responsible for selecting and determining the correct dosage to achieve the desirable effects of conscious sedation and analgesia. The RN is responsible for the administration of conscious sedation and analgesia medication(s) and for monitoring the patient. The RN must be knowledgeable about the pharmacologic aspects of each medication administered, including the expected action, normal pediatric dosage, possible adverse effects, and available reversal agents.

Although the physician is responsible for determining the dosage, the RN who administers the medication is also legally liable. Therefore the RN must be able to determine if the dosage is safe for the pediatric patient. A variety of formulas are used to determine pediatric medication dosage (e.g., Young's rule, Clark's rule). However, these formulas determine pediatric dosages in relation to standard adult dosage and often are inaccurate. The most reliable and accurate method for determining medication dosage for the pediatric patient is body surface area (Figure 8-1).

1. Clark's rule:

$$\text{Estimated child's dosage} = \frac{\text{Weight (lb) of child}}{150\ \text{lb}} \times \text{Adult dosage}$$

2. Body surface calculation:

$$\text{Estimated child's dosage} = \frac{\text{Surface area of child (m}^2)}{1.7\ \text{m}^2} \times \text{Adult dosage}$$

Oral Sedation

Oral sedation offers advantages over other routes because it is essentially painless and is convenient to administer. Care must be taken to measure the dosage accurately. The plastic disposable syringe offers the most accurate method for measuring small pediatric dosages. It may also serve as a convenient vehicle for administering the medication. When administering the medication, the RN should place the syringe tip along the side of the mouth and slowly squirt the medicine toward the buccal vestibule, not toward the throat. Medications that are bitter are often mixed with popsicle syrup, juice, or flavored syrups.

Intramuscular Sedation

Intramuscular (IM) sedation is less frequently used because of the discomfort caused to the patient and the lack of predictability of the sedative level. Children are frightened by the mere thought of receiving a "shot" and would rather endure the pain of their disease or injury (Eland & Anderson, 1977). However, there are instances in which oral sedation has little effect on behavior, the patient is uncooperative, and other techniques for sedation are ruled out; in such cases IM sedation may be used.

The preferred IM injection sites for children include the vastus lateralis, ventrogluteal, dorsogluteal, and deltoid (Table 8-3). Medications from a glass ampule should be drawn up with a filtered needle to prevent injecting small fragments of glass.

Rectal Sedation

Rectal sedation is often used for the patient who is unable to take medication by mouth. One major disadvantage of this method is that the level of sedation is unpredictable. For example, absorption of the medication is delayed if stool is present.

The suppository is administered by gently inserting it into the rectum, beyond the rectal sphincter. If the child expels the suppository, it may be reinserted by gently

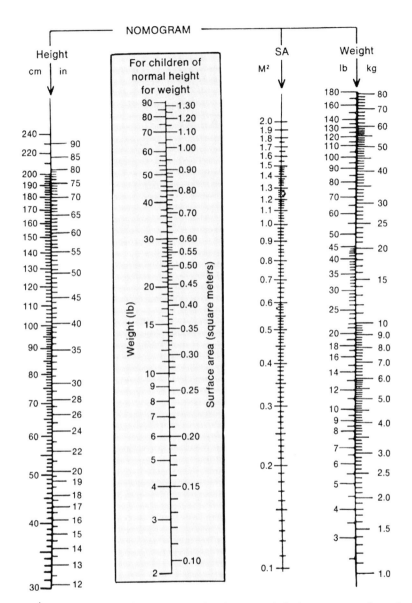

FIGURE 8-1 | West nomogram (for estimation of surface areas). Surface area is indicated where a straight line connecting height and weight intersects surface area (SA) column, or if patient is roughly of normal proportion, from weight alone (enclosed area). (Nomogram modified from data of E. Boyd by C. D. West; from Behrman, R. E., & Vaughan, V. C. [Eds.]. [1996]. *Nelson textbook of pediatrics* [15th ed.]. Philadelphia: W. B. Saunders.)

TABLE 8-3 *Intramuscular Injection Sites in Children*

SITE	DISCUSSION

VASTUS LATERALIS

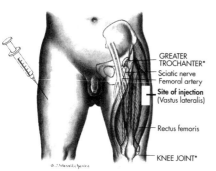

LOCATION

Palpate to find greater trochanter and knee joints; divide vertical distance between these two landmarks into quadrants; inject into middle of upper quadrant

NEEDLE INSERTION

Insert needle at 45-degree angle toward knee in infants and in young children or needle perpendicular to thigh or slightly angled toward anterior thigh

ADVANTAGES

Large, well-developed muscle that can tolerate larger quantities of fluid

No important nerves or blood vessels in this location

Easily accessible if child is supine, side-lying, or sitting

A tourniquet can be applied above injection site to delay drug hypersensitivity reaction if necessary

DISADVANTAGES

Thrombosis of femoral artery from injection in midthigh area

Sciatic nerve damage from long needle injected posteriorly and medially into small extremity

VENTROGLUTEAL

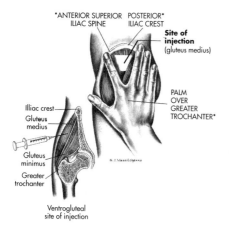

LOCATION

Palpate to locate greater trochanter, anterior superior iliac tubercle (found by flexing thigh at hip and measuring up to 1 to 2 cm above crease formed in groin), and posterior iliac crest; place palm of hand over greater trochanter, index finger over anterior superior iliac tubercle, and middle finger along crest of ilium posteriorly as far as possible; inject into center of V formed by fingers

NEEDLE INSERTION

Insert needle perpendicular to site but angled slightly toward iliac crest

ADVANTAGES

Free of important nerves and vascular structures

Easily identified by prominent bony landmarks

Thinner layer of subcutaneous tissue than in dorsogluteal site, thus less chance of depositing drug subcutaneously rather than intramuscularly

Easily accessible if child is supine, prone, or side-lying

Less painful than vastus lateralis

DISADVANTAGES

Health professionals' unfamiliarity with site

Not suitable for use of a tourniquet

From Wong, D. L. (1997). *Whaley & Wong's Essentials of pediatric nursing* (5th ed., pp. 716-717). St. Louis: Mosby.

DORSOGLUTEAL

*POSTERIOR SUPERIOR
ILIAC SPINE
*Gluteus medius
Site of injection
(gluteus maximus)

Sciatic nerve
GREATER TROCHANTER
OF FEMUR

G. J. Wassilchenko

LOCATION

Locate greater trochanter and posterior superior iliac spine; draw imaginary line between these two points and inject lateral and superior to line into gluteus muscle

NEEDLE INSERTION

Insert needle perpendicular to surface on which child is lying when prone

ADVANTAGES

In older child large muscle mass; well-developed muscle can tolerate greater volume of fluid

Child does not see needle and syringe

Easily accessible if child is prone or side-lying

DISADVANTAGES

Contraindicted in children who have not been walking for at least 1 year

Danger of injury to sciatic nerve

Thick, subcutaneous fat, predisposing to deposition of drug subcutaneously rather than intramuscularly

Not suitable for use of a tourniquet

Inaccessible if child is supine

Exposure of site may cause embarrassment in older child

DELTOID

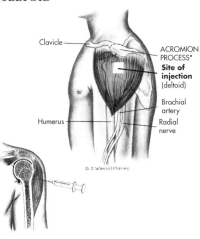

Clavicle

ACROMION
PROCESS*
**Site of
injection**
(deltoid)

Brachial
artery
Humerus
Radial
nerve

G. J. Wassilchenko

LOCATION

Locate acromion process; inject only into upper third of muscle that begins about 2 finger-breadths below acromion

NEEDLE INSERTION

Insert needle perpendicular to site but angled slightly toward shoulder

ADVANTAGES

Faster absorption rates than gluteal sites

Tourniquet can be applied above injection site

Easily accessible with minimum removal of clothing

DISADVANTAGES

Small muscle mass; only limited amounts of drug can be injected

Small margins of safety with possible damage to radial nerve

Pain with repeated injections

taping or holding the buttocks together until the urge to expel the contents passes. If the dosage ordered is less than 1 suppository, it is recommended that the suppository not be cut because of its irregular shape and the difficulty in determining the precise measurement of medication.

Intravenous Administration

Intravenous (IV) administration allows for titration of medication to the desired patient response. The most common sites selected for IV sedation in pediatric patients are the superficial veins in the hand, wrist, or arm. Because venipuncture is painful and frightening to the pediatric patient, distraction techniques should be used. EMLA 5%, a eutectic mixture of local anesthetics, may be applied to the site to provide analgesia before venipuncture. To achieve optimal effects, the EMLA should be applied to the potential site(s) 60 minutes before puncture (Halperin et al., 1989). An appropriate period of time should be allowed for full evaluation of the effects of the medication on the patient. Hammer (1992) suggests waiting 10 minutes before administering a second dose via the IV route.

The IV administration may be started with a butterfly catheter, IV catheter, or heparin lock. Fluids should always be administered in a drip control chamber or burette to prevent fluid overload. Pediatric IV administration sets are calibrated to flow at 60 drops per milliliter (60 gtt/ml).

Commonly Administered Medications

Nursing staff should be educated about the proper administration of all medications that are approved by the institution for pediatric sedation. Table 8-4 lists doses of medications commonly used for pediatric sedation. This list is only a guide. Consideration should be given to the type of procedure, age of the child, weight, anxiety level, desired level of sedation, and route options for the particular medication.

CONCLUSION

The RN responsible for the management of the pediatric patient scheduled for sedation and analgesia should be aware of the child's age and weight and should have predetermined the appropriate medication dosage ranges before administering any medication. Many institutions have a separate standard of care for the administration of pediatric sedation that includes detailed guidelines for the nonanesthesia provider during the administration of pediatric sedation and analgesia (Figure 8-2).

TABLE 8-4 *Medication List*		
DRUG	ROUTE	DOSE (mg/kg)
Barbiturates		
Methohexital	Rectal	20-30
	Intramuscular	10
Thiopental	Rectal	20-30
	Intramuscular	10
Benzodiazepines		
Diazepam	Oral	0.1-0.3
	Intravenous	0.1-0.3
	Intramuscular	Not recommended
	Rectal	0.2-0.3
Midazolam	Oral	0.5-0.75
	Intravenous	0.05-0.15
	Intramuscular	0.05-0.15
	Rectal	0.5-0.75
	Nasal	0.2-0.5
	Sublingual	0.2-0.5
Ketamine	Oral	3-10
	Intravenous	1-3
	Intramuscular	2-10
	Rectal	5-10
	Nasal	3-5
	Sublingual	3-5
Opioids		
Morphine	Intravenous	0.1-0.3
	Intramuscular	0.1-0.3
	Rectal	Not recommended
Meperidine	Intravenous	1-3
	Intramuscular	1-3
	Rectal	Not recommended
Fentanyl	Oral transmucosal	0.015-0.020 (15-20 µg)
	Sublingual	0.010-0.015 (10-15 µg)
	Intravenous	0.001-0.005 (1-5 µg/kg in increments of 0.5-1.0 µg/kg)

From Coté, C. J. (1994). Sedation for the pediatric patient: A review. *Pediatric Clinics of North America, 41*(1), 45.

Holmes Regional Medical Center, Inc. (HMRC)
Melbourne, Florida
Care of the Pediatric Conscious Sedation Patient

Objective: To provide all pediatric patients (under 18 years of age) receiving depressive sedation for diagnostic or therapeutic procedures a like standard of care, regardless of where the care is rendered in the medical center. The monitoring and care may be exceeded at any time, based on the judgment of the responsible physician.

POLICY

A. This policy covers patients cared for in all of the following areas:
   - Critical care units
   - Developmental intervention unit
   - Electroencephalography
   - Emergency departments (see exception U below)
   - Endoscopy labs
   - Holmes Regional Ambulatory Surgery Center
   - Hyperbarics (see exception S below)
   - Medical imaging
   - Magnetic resonance imaging (see exception T below)
   - Neonatal intensive care unit
   - Palm Bay Community Hospital
   - Palm Bay Surgery Center
   - Pediatrics
B. Conscious sedation is characterized by these elements:
   1. Depressed consciousness
   2. Independent airway
   3. Responsiveness to verbal stimuli
   4. Presence of protective reflexes
   5. Amnesia

C. This policy is not intended to cover deep sedation.

   Deep sedation is defined by the American Academy of Pediatrics as "a medically controlled state of unconsciousness from which the patient is not easily aroused. It may be accompanied by a partial or complete loss of protective reflexes, and includes the inability to maintain a patent airway independently and respond purposefully to physical stimulation or verbal command. Deep sedation and general anesthesia are virtually inseparable for monitoring purposes. The distinction is made in the pediatric population to describe appropriate levels of monitoring. It may be administered only by an anesthesiologist.

D. A registered nurse may administer the medications and must have successfully completed the following:
   1. PALS is recommended.
   — or —
   2. BLS with annual recertification.
   3. Training in the recognition of the cardiovascular and respiratory side effects of sedatives, as well as the variability and unique aspects of pediatric response. Training in airway management is also required.
   4. Recertification is required; PALS is recommended.
   5. Successful completion of a basic dysrhythmia class is also mandatory.

FIGURE 8-2 | Sample standard of care for the pediatric patient receiving conscious sedation and analgesia. *ACT,* Activated clotting time; *BLS,* basic life support; *IM,* intramuscularly; *IV,* intravenous; *NPO,* nothing by mouth; *NTE,* not to exceed; *PALS,* pathology and laboratory studies; *PO,* by mouth; *PRN,* as required; *PT/PTT,* prothrombin time/partial thromboplastin time; *SC,* subcutaneously. (Courtesy Holmes Regional Medical Center, Inc.)

6. The person administering the drugs must be knowledgeable of the pharmacology of the drugs administered as evidenced by completing the required class on the agents and passing a posttest. Loading doses may be given by the nurse under the direction of and in the presence of the physician. (See Appendix I for Outline of Pharmacology Inservice.)
E. Preprocedural testing is performed as indicated by the patient's clinical status and medical history with the exception of a PT/PTT being required for patients undergoing an elective procedure who are receiving anticoagulants. ACT testing may be substituted.
F. A pediatric patient who has received any type of sedation must be transported by a nurse or technologist who meets the educational criteria listed in D above.
G. A licensed nurse or qualified member of the medical staff will be present whose primary responsibility will be to monitor the patient during the procedure. This cannot be the person performing the actual procedure.
H. Patients for IV sedation are recommended to be NPO for 3 hours except during emergent situations.
I. The medications that may be used as conscious sedative agents are:
   1. Chloral hydrate
   2. Versed
   3. Narcotics (morphine, Demerol, or fentanyl)
   4. Ketamine, propofol, brevetrol, and ultra–short-acting narcotics should be used only by an anesthesiologist.
   5. Muscle relaxants are contraindicated.
J. Suggested dosing guidelines for pediatric patients are:
   1. Chloral hydrate: 100 mg/kg for the first 10 kg; 50 mg/kg thereafter. Maximum dose: 2000 mg. Up to half of the original dose may be repeated after 30-45 minutes if initial dose is inadequate. If still ineffective, exam will be rescheduled.
      a. All orders written for chloral hydrate should be written as the total milligram dose, not the volume of the drug to be administered (i.e., 750 mg followed by 500 mg if needed [NOT 1½ tsp followed by 1 tsp if needed]).
      b. Children should be dosed on kilogram weight, not on pound weight, not to exceed 2 g. It should be kept in mind that the maximum adult dose is 2 g.
   2. Versed 0.5-1.0 mg/kg NTE 15 mg po in 10-12 ml in grape juice is a preferred oral premedication.
   3. Versed: 0.1-0.2 mg/kg IV. Maximum dose: NTE 2.5 mg.
   4. Morphine: 0.1-0.2 mg/kg; NTE 15 mg dose.
   5. Demerol: 1-2 mg/kg IV. (Maximum dose: 100 mg.)
   6. Titration to desired effect is the preferred method of administration, instead of fixed dosing schedules, recognizing that these doses are needed to achieve the desired end point.
   7. Pediatric patients require decreased dosages and are more susceptible to rebound effects than are adults.
K. Suggested additional dosage guidelines for children:
   1. 0.02 mg/kg for Versed IV q 5 min PRN for agitation.
   2. 0.1 mg/kg for morphine IV q 5 min PRN for agitation.
   3. 1 mg/kg for Demerol IV q 5 min PRN for agitation.
   4. Titration to desired effect is the preferred method of administration rather than fixed dosing schedules.
   5. Different dosage schedules may be appropriate for children during certain procedures.
   6. Pediatric patients require decreased dosages and are more susceptible to rebound effects than are adults.
L. Suggested dosage guidelines for continuous infusions of sedative agents are:
   1. 0.4 mcg/kg/min Versed (0.4 mcg/kg/hr).
   2. If sedation is inadequate, the rate may be titrated to desired effect.
   3. Different dosage schedules may be appropriate for children during certain procedures.
   4. Pediatric patients require decreased dosages and are more susceptible to rebound effects than are older patients.

FIGURE 8-2 cont'd | For legend see opposite page.

M. Antagonist drugs must be immediately available:
1. Naloxone (Narcan) is the agent of choice for reversal of either narcotic sedation or combined narcotic/benzodiazepine sedation. (<20 kg = 0.01-0.10 mg/kg IV/IM/SC q 3-5 min PRN). (≥20 kg = ([>5 yr of age]) = 2 mg dose IV/IM/SC q 3-5 min PRN).
2. Flumazenil (Romazicon) is the agent of choice for pure benzodiazepine sedation (0.01 mg/kg).
N. An emergency kit or standard emergency cart must be readily available, which will stock the necessary drugs and equipment appropriate for the flow rate required to resuscitate a nonbreathing and unconscious patient and provide continuous support.
O. Suction and oxygen will be available at the bedside.
P. A secure IV access is maintained in the presence of IV sedation.
Q. Documentation of the following will be kept:
1. Drug(s) used
2. Amount of drug administered
3. Time of drug administration
4. Values of the various monitored parameters recorded at 5-minute intervals
5. Signature of person administering drugs
6. Signature of person monitoring patient
R. The standard of care is attached to this policy and is maintained in the HRMC *Operations Manual.*
S. The hyperbarics unit monitors only cardiac rhythm, pulse, and respirations while the patient is in the chamber because of safety issues. (Pulse oximeters and BP equipment are not available for use in the chamber.)
T. MRI monitors only pulse oximeters while the patient is in the chamber because of safety issues.
U. The emergency departments may opt not to monitor blood pressures every 5 minutes if the child is very agitated or restless.
V. Performance improvement (PI) monitoring and evaluation will be performed by each department as detailed in Appendix II.

PROCEDURE
I. PATIENT EDUCATION
A. The nurse, technologist, or technician will ensure that each outpatient and the parent/guardian will receive an individualized instruction sheet.
B. Patient-specific information relating to the patient's condition or physician's orders will be added as needed.
II. PHYSIOLOGICAL FUNCTIONING
A. The **nurse** will administer the drugs as ordered by the physician.
The **nurse, technologist,** or **technician** will:
B. Obtain and document preprocedural vital signs to include: blood pressure (BP), heart rate (HR), respiratory rate (RR), temperature (T), and a baseline oxygen saturation determination (SaO_2).
C. Monitor cardiac rhythm, and document BP, HR, and SaO_2 q 5 min during the procedure, or more frequently as indicated by the patient's condition or physician's order.
D. Patients receiving continuous infusions require continuous SaO_2 and cardiac monitoring. BP, HR, and RR must be documented at least q 30 min.
E. Administer low-flow oxygen (2-3 L/min) therapy during the actual procedure via nasal cannula as warranted by patient's condition to maintain the oxygen level ≥ the preprocedural level. The fraction of inspired oxygen (FiO_2) rate may be increased as indicated by the patient's condition. Oxygen is very safe to give at 2-3 L/min; its use should be strongly considered by the physician and given whenever possible.
F. Continue cardiac and oxygen monitoring postprocedure only as indicated by patient's condition or per physician's order.
G. Monitor and document BP, HR, RR, and SaO_2 q 15 min x 4 and/or per patient's clinical status or physician's order.

FIGURE 8-2 cont'd | For legend see p. 154.

III. PREVENTION OF COMPLICATIONS/SAFETY

The nurse, technologist, or technician will:

A. Notify physician of any deterioration in patient's mental or clinical status.
B. Institute and document the appropriate interventions for significant findings.
C. Report any significant changes to the physician.
D. Evaluate and document patient responses to the interventions.
E. Monitor the patient's temperature postprocedure, as indicated by the patient's condition or per physician's order.
F. Monitor the patient's BP, HR, and RR, and SaO_2 q 15 min x 4 and/or per patient's clinical status or physician's order.
G. Keep siderails up constantly while patient is on a stretcher/crib unattended by staff.
H. Assure that patients are assisted from stretcher/wheelchair.
I. Assure that wheels are locked on stretcher/crib and wheelchair at all times, except during transport.
J. Label IV additives per hospital policy.
K. Assist patients who have received other than local anesthesia to car; use of a wheelchair is required.

IV. PAIN MANAGEMENT/COMFORT

The nurse will:

A. Administer analgesics per departmental policy or physician order.

The nurse, technologist, or technician will:

A. Apply blankets as requested or as indicated by patient's condition.
B. Assess the patient's response to pain.
C. Document patient's response to interventions.

V. DISCHARGE/TRANSFER PLANNING

The nurse, technologist, or technician will:

A. Determine that the patient meets the following criteria:
  1. Cardiovascular function and airway patency are satisfactory and stable.
  2. Patient is easily arousable, and protective reflexes are intact.
  3. Patient can talk (if age appropriate).
  4. Patient can sit up unaided (if age appropriate).
  5. In a very young, or handicapped, child incapable of the usually expected responses, the presedation level of responsiveness or a level as close as possible to the normal level for that child has been achieved.
  6. The state of hydration is adequate.
B. Determine that a physician's discharge order is present.
C. Give the instruction sheet to the responsible adult.
D. Obtain the signature of the patient/significant other after they verbalize understanding of the instructions.
E. Place a copy of the instructions in the medical record.
F. Give a comprehensive report to the receiving nurse or designee.

Developed: 11/93
Revised: 12/93; 01/94; 03/94; 09/6/94; 09/12/94
Approved: 10/94
Marge Miller, RN, MSN, CCRN
pedsf.ivs

FIGURE 8-2 cont'd | For legend see p. 154.

REFERENCES

American Academy of Pediatrics. (1992). Guidelines for monitoring and management of pediatric patients during and after sedation for diagnostic and therapeutic procedures. *Pediatrics, 89*(6), 1110.

American Nurses Association. (1991). *Position statement on the role of the registered nurse (RN) in the management of patients receiving IV conscious sedation for short-term therapeutic, diagnostic, or surgical procedures.* Kansas City: Author.

Association of Operating Room Nurses. (1997). Recommended practices: Monitoring the patient receiving IV conscious sedation. In *AORN Standards and Recommended Practices*. Denver: Author.

Coté, C. J. (1994). NPO after midnight for children: A reappraisal. *Anesthesiology, 72,* 589-592.

Eland, J. M., & Anderson, J. E. (1977). The experience of pain in children. In A. K. Jacox, (Ed.), *Pain: A source book for nurses and other health professionals* (pp. 453-473). Boston: Little, Brown.

Halperin, D. L., Koren, G., Attias, D., Pellegrini, E., Greenberg, M. L., & Wyss, M. (1989). Topical skin anesthesia for venous, subcutaneous drug reservoir and lumbar punctures in children. *Pediatrics, 84*(2), 281-284.

Hammer, S. J. (1992). Pediatric update: Conscious sedation for infants and children in the emergency department. *Journal of Emergency Nursing, 18*(2), 165-166.

Holzman, R. S., Cullen D. J., Eichhorn, H. H., & Philip, J. H. (1994). Guidelines for sedation by nonanesthesiologist during diagnostic and therapeutic procedures. *Journal of Clinical Anesthesiology, 6,* 265-276.

U. S. Department of Health and Human Services. (Feb. 1992). *Acute pain management: Operative or medical procedures and trauma* (AHCPR Pub. No. 92-0032). Rockville, MD: Acute Pain Management Guideline Panel, Agency for Health Care Policy and Research, Public Health Service.

Yaster, M., Nichols, D. G., Deshpande, J. K., & Wetzel, R. C. (1990). Midazolam-fentanyl intravenous sedation in children: Case report of respiratory arrest. *Pediatrics, 86*(3), 463-466.

BIBLIOGRAPHY

American College of Emergency Physicians. (1993). The use of pediatric sedation and analgesia. *Annals of Emergency Medicine, 22,* 626-627.

American Academy of Pediatrics, Committee on Drugs. (1988). Emergency drug doses for infants and children. *Pediatrics, 81,* 462-465.

Sedation in the Mechanically Ventilated Patient

There are many indications for the administration of sedation and analgesia to the critically ill patient; however, this chapter will focus on the assessment and interventions for agitation and delirium as a means of determining the need for and patient outcomes related to sedation and analgesia. The RN will be able to identify risk factors for agitation and delirium, describe interventions aimed at correcting conditions that precipitate agitation and delirium, and address pharmacologic and nonpharmacologic measures that are an integral part of management in the critically ill patient.

Critically ill patients who require mechanical ventilation often have high levels of anxiety and discomfort. Some studies of intensive care units (ICU) have reported patient symptoms ranging from severe anxiety to excruciating pain. Many patients show signs of restlessness and delirium (Crippen, 1994; Geary, 1994; Harvey, 1996; & Riker, Gilles, & Cox, 1994). Many critically ill patients are not able to express their level of discomfort, either because of the disease process or prescribed medications (i.e., anxiolytics, analgesics, neuromuscular blocking agents). In caring for these patients, the RN often relies on signs and symptoms of agitation and delirium (e.g., restlessness, anxiety, and fear) to modify the plan of care as appropriate. There is evidence that morbidity and mortality rates are higher among agitated patients, so prompt identification and management of agitation is essential for achieving positive patient outcomes (Murray, 1994; Riker, Gilles, & Cox, 1994; Shelly, 1994; & Stern, 1994).

Patient discomfort in the ICU takes on many forms; foremost among these are dyspnea and pain. Intubated patients are likely to have varying degrees of dyspnea that may result from impaired gas exchange (e.g., pulmonary disorder) or other disorders that prevent the delivery of oxygen to the cells (e.g., cardiogenic shock, severe anemia). If an adequate supply of oxygen is not readily provided to the cells, the acutely dyspneic patient's psychologic coping mechanisms may quickly break down to a state of panic and urgent flight behavior (Jensen & Justic, 1995). Immediate interventions should be aimed at correcting the oxygen deficit and may include adjusting positive pressure ventilation, increasing the percentage of delivered oxygen, and administering bronchodilators as ordered.

Pain is a noxious sensation that elicits an immediate urge to withdraw from the source. There are multiple causes of pain that the patient may experience (e.g., surgical incision site, chest tubes, arterial-venous punctures, ischemia to limbs or internal organs). Pain, whether continual, intermittent, or episodic, elicits a fear response, which exacerbates the patient's underlying anxiety.

One of the roles of the RN is to relieve the underlying causes of pain and discomfort by direct intervention. For example, in the case of dyspnea the intervention may include clearing the airway of secretions, adjusting the ventilatory parameters, or administering bronchial dilators. If deterioration of the other systems, such as pump failure, is the cause of the dyspnea, the symptoms will not be eliminated until the underlying abnormality is corrected. Additional interventions may include the administration of analgesics and antianxiety agents (i.e., anxiolytics), assessing their efficacy, and providing nonpharmacologic measures such as therapeutic touch, patient and family education, and reassurance.

When the sensation of dyspnea, anxiety, or pain is not effectively managed, the symptoms exert a powerful negative impact on several organs. The motor activity can exhaust the patient's already-limited ability to deliver adequate oxygen and nutrition to the cells. The agitated patient tends to resist the mechanical ventilation, sometimes to the point of biting the endotracheal tube and occluding it. The resultant deterioration in oxygen delivery exacerbates the patient's sense of dyspnea and heightens the agitation. Persistent anxiety, pain, and dyspnea coupled with major hemodynamic or metabolic disturbance can cause the patient's agitation to progress to an acute confusional state. This condition affects as many as 50% of all adult ICU patients (Crippen, 1994; Harvey, 1996; & Luer, 1995).

Delirium, sometimes called ICU psychosis, is now understood to be a reversible organic syndrome. Current research suggests that, when a critically ill patient becomes agitated and confused, the condition is due primarily to dysfunction of brain metabolism related to abnormal neurotransmission (Crippen, 1994; Geary, 1994; & Harvey, 1996); and it has a broad range of unwanted consequences.

Unlike other organs, the brain depends on a constant supply of glucose and oxygen. Interruption in the delivery of these vital nutrients quickly disrupts the delicate chemistry of the brain. Many disease processes affecting the critically ill patient impair glucose and oxygen transport to the brain, whereas other abnormalities, such as drug toxicity or high ammonia levels, directly alter neurotransmission.

When an adult patient who complains of chest pain is encountered, the RN may initially entertain a diagnosis of acute myocardial infarction. In the same manner, the nurse in the ICU must learn to consider a diagnosis of acute brain dysfunction when the patient becomes agitated or delirious. This interpretation of agitation encourages the RN to assess for deteriorating organ systems and to appraise the patient's level of discomfort and confusion.

PATHOPHYSIOLOGIC MECHANISMS OF AGITATION AND DELIRIUM

Excessive, uncontrolled, or irrational motor activity, heightened autonomic discharge, and internal tension (Crippen, 1994; Geary, 1994; Riker, Gilles, & Cox, 1994) characterize agitation in the critically ill patient. Agitation manifests itself in the patient pulling on tubes, side rails, or bed sheets; thrashing in the bed; and fighting against the ventilator rather than breathing with it.

In its early stages agitation is characterized by restlessness, difficulty sleeping, and a short attention span (Crippen & Ermakov, 1992). Psychologic coping mechanisms are eroded, and the patient exhibits a diminished tolerance of uncomfortable procedures, such as turning or suctioning the airway.

If the agitation progresses, neurologic assessment reveals symptoms of global cognitive impairment (Geary, 1994; & Harvey, 1996). The patient becomes unable to process information rationally or to retain information for more than a few minutes. The patient may require vigorous verbal and tactile stimulation to get his/her attention and is likely to soon forget instructions or information. Other neurologic abnormalities associated with agitation include alternating periods of hyperalertness and lethargy, which are virtually diagnostic of this syndrome (Crippen, 1994). The characteristics of agitation and delirium are summarized in Box 9-1. At first the patient is confused as to time. If the condition worsens, the confusion extends to place and eventually to person as well. If the delirium continues, it may result in coma.

With poor coordination and short-term memory deficit, the patient may have difficulty writing a complete sentence in answer to questioning. Sometimes the patient cannot write his/her full name, faltering after making the first few letters and then losing track of the goal. Often the patient is unable to lie still or sleep unless given sedatives or neuroleptics. The patient may heed a command to "Lie still!" for a time but moments later may strain to reach the endotracheal tube despite clear, firm instructions to the contrary.

Agitation was once considered a psychologic response to the stress of major illness and admission to the ICU. It is now known to be a reversible organic syndrome related to dysfunction of the brain. It differs from true psychosis in several ways. First, a functional psychosis is not known to have an organic cause (American Psychiatric Association, 1996; Crippen & Ermakov, 1992; & Geary, 1994). Second, functional psychosis usually has an internal consistency, whereas those with delirium

---

BOX 9-1 *Characteristics of Delirium in Critically Ill Patient*

1. Acute onset caused by impaired brain metabolism
2. Globally impaired cognitive function
3. Excessive uncontrolled motor activity
4. Attention deficit and impaired short-term memory
5. Alternating restlessness and lethargy
6. Disrupted sleep/wake cycle
7. Increased autonomic discharge

exhibit fragmented thoughts. The psychotic individual may have bizarre ideas, but the ideas are for the most part consistent and logical within that frame of reference. Psychotic and delirious patients may have hallucinations and paranoid ideas, and both may have delusions, which are fixed, illogical beliefs that are not responsive to conflicting evidence (American Psychiatric Association, 1996). Third, the delirium of the patient with impaired brain metabolism is more global than that of the functional psychotic. Memory and attention span are diminished, and there is disruption of the sleep-wake cycle. In some cases the excessive release of neurotransmitters will prevent the ICU patient from sleeping for several days.

Some researchers suggest that preexisting personality disorders can contribute to the ICU patient's agitation and delirium (Geary, 1994; & Harvey, 1996). Individuals who have obsessive compulsive disorders may have high levels of anxiety because of their restricted movements. Patients who have a strong need to control others may decompensate in the ICU environment, where caregivers take charge of the patient's every function.

Perhaps the most striking symptoms that set the delirious, critically ill patient apart from the functional psychotic one are the musculoskeletal abnormalities seen in critical care. These patients exhibit tremors, rigidity, hyperreflexia, uncoordinated movements, and disequilibrium. These signs are not commonly associated with the outpatient schizophrenic or delusional person.

Two mechanisms produce neurologic abnormalities in the critically ill patient. The first is the impact of prolonged states of apprehension and discomfort, especially dyspnea and pain, on the brain. The second mechanism involves the hemodynamic and metabolic disorders that affect critically ill patients (Box 9-2).

Brain Function

In addition to its autonomic regulatory functions, the central nervous system processes sensory input and channels it to higher regions of the brain, where it is interpreted against past experience (Crippen & Ermakov, 1992). At the same time the brain supplies emotional response to the data, which affects the intensity of the experience and the response.

The brain disregards 99% of the sensory input it receives. It selects significant input and channels it through neuronal circuits to the appropriate motor and cognitive centers in the cortex. These centers then send out appropriate responses through the motor axis and cerebellum, producing purposeful, coordinated actions.

The emotional response to the sensory input depends on its comparison with previous experience. For example, the sight of a snake in the grass usually elicits an immediate fear response. The brain releases a surge of catecholamines and coricotropin-releasing factor, which prepare the body for fight or flight. If the perceiver decides that the snake is harmless, the emotional response abates with the release of other inhibiting transmitters, such as γ-aminobutyric acid (GABA), and emotional equilibrium is restored.

BOX 9-2 *Subjective and Objective Factors That Impair Brain Function*

SUBJECTIVE FACTORS

Dyspnea
Pain
Anxiety
Nausea, thirst, hunger
Diarrhea, urinary incontinence
Preexisting psychopathology
Intense sensory input
Sleep deprivation

OBJECTIVE FACTORS

Increased production of:
Norepinephrine
Dopamine
β-Endorphins
Corticotropin-releasing factor
Decreased production of:
Intraneural enzymes that return
transmitters to producing neurons

HEMODYNAMIC AND METABOLIC DISORDERS

Intrinsic to brain
Stroke
Increased intracranial pressure caused
by trauma

Space-occupying lesions
Meningitis
Toxoplasmosis
Withdrawal from addictive substances
Extrinsic to brain
Hypoxemia
Hypercapnia
Hypotension/shock
Hypoglycemia
Electrolyte imbalance
Acid-base imbalance
Drug toxicity
Renal or liver failure

NEUROLOGIC SIGNS/SYMPTOMS OF BRAIN DYSFUNCTION

Global mental impairment
Alternating hyperalertness and lethargy
Loss of short-term memory
Uncontrolled motor activity
Tremulousness, musculoskeletal rigidity
Disorientation
Delusions and hallucinations
Paranoid ideation
Coma

Prolonged periods of apprehension elicit an increased production of norepinephrine from central structures, principally the locus coeruleus. High levels of norepinephrine produce anxiety, restlessness, and inability to sleep and impair the brain's ability to filter out unwanted sensory input. As a result, ICU patients lose their ability to discriminate, which heightens anxiety or agitation (Harvey, 1996).

The patient's subjective state is similar to the condition that follows ingesting a cold remedy containing ephedrine, a sympathomimetic, at bedtime. The resulting state of restlessness, palpitations, and inability to sleep is due to the stimulating effects of the catecholamine analog and is similar to the experience of the ICU patient. Unrelieved pain and hypoxia elicit similar outflows of catecholamines and produce even more pronounced stress on cerebral metabolism.

In response to the continued sympathetic discharge, the cerebral cortex becomes exhausted (Barber, 1995; Crippen, 1994; & Geary, 1994). The brain's resources, which are likely to be already compromised, are further taxed and its ability to metabolize nutrients is impaired.

It is important to remember that an anxious patient who becomes restless, irritable, and unable to sleep may be demonstrating the early warning signs of impending brain dysfunction. This condition warrants immediate assessment of all organ systems and laboratory values to determine the causative agent.

Brain metabolism is also impaired by hemodynamic and metabolic disorders, which commonly affect critically ill patients (Box 9-3). Disorders that are intrinsic to the brain may include stroke, space-occupying lesions, and swelling resulting from trauma, hydrocephalus, or infection.

A number of hemodynamic and metabolic disease processes extrinsic to the brain alter its metabolism. Common examples are hypoxemia, hypotension, and hypoglycemia. Hypoxemia, a state of low partial pressure of oxygen in the blood, may develop from pulmonary disorders such as bronchospasm, pneumonia, pulmonary effusions, or pulmonary emboli (Bizek, 1995). Disorders such as asthma or cancer of the lung may also lead to decreased gas exchange and lowered blood oxygen levels.

Mechanical problems with the ventilator or endotracheal tube may impede oxygen delivery. An inadequately inflated endotracheal balloon or dislodgment of the endotracheal tube will compromise oxygen delivery. A decrease in peak airway pressure may also stem from leaks in the ventilator tubing or an improperly sealed cap or nebulizer. Any of these problems may make the patient severely agitated as a result of a rapidly falling blood oxygen level. Any persistent low-oxygen state impedes brain metabolism and disrupts neurotransmission.

Hypotension caused by pump failure, sepsis, anaphylaxis, or hemorrhage impairs the delivery of oxygen to and removal of carbon dioxide from the brain. Even if the lung is able to exchange gases at the alveolar-capillary interface, the organs do not receive a sufficient blood supply for cellular respiration. Acidosis accompanying hypotension further degrades brain metabolism.

Hypoglycemia rapidly disrupts brain metabolism, setting off a cascade of injury, which alters neurotransmission, and the rediffusion of transmitters back into the producing cells. Dopamine surges from the limbic system cause widespread disruption of cerebral and lower regions of the brain (Barber, 1995).

Other metabolic disorders that disrupt brain function include metabolic acidosis; elevated blood urea nitrogen (BUN), creatinine, and ammonia levels; and hyponatremia. Reaction to one of many medications commonly administered in the ICU may contribute to agitation. Steroids are a well-known cause of confusion. H_2 blockers, antibiotics, bronchodilators, and antihistamines have also been linked to agitation and confusion (Crippen & Ermakov, 1992; Geary, 1994; Harvey, 1996; & Luer, 1995).

Withdrawal from opiates, sedatives, antidepressants, alcohol, or tobacco can cause agitation and confusion. Forms of substance abuse may be overlooked in the ICU when the focus is on major organ failure. Not infrequently, tobacco addiction

BOX 9-3 *Hemodynamic and Metabolic Causes of Agitation and Confusion*

HEMODYNAMIC

Impaired cerebral perfusion caused by cerebral vascular accident, tumor, increased intracranial pressure

Meningitis, toxoplasmosis

Anoxic encephalopathy

Hypotension caused by sepsis or cardiogenic, anaphylactic, or hemorrhagic shock

METABOLIC

Hypoglycemia

Acidosis

Hyponatremia

Elevated blood urea nitrogen and creatinine levels

Elevated serum ammonia levels

Myxedema

Corticosteroid insufficiency

DRUG EFFECTS

Antihistamines

Anticholinergics

Corticosteroids

Digitalis

H_2 antagonists

Impipenem, penicillin, amphotericin B, cephalosporins

Lidocaine, procainamide, quinidine, propranolol

Nitroprusside

Metoclopramide

Nonsteroidal antiinflammatory drugs

Theophylline

DRUG WITHDRAWAL

Opiates, cocaine, alcohol

Exogenous steroids

Tranquilizers

Antidepressants

Amphetamines

Data from Crippen, D. (1994). *Critical Care Nurse Quarterly, 16*(4), 80-95; Geary, S. (1994). *Critical Care Nursing Quarterly, 17*(1), 51-63; Harvey, M. (1996). *American Journal of Critical Care, 5*(1), 7-15.

contributes to a patient's anxiety and agitation. Use of a nicotine patch often alleviates a significant part of the patient's discomfort and allows for lower doses of anxiolytics.

Alcohol withdrawal, a familiar syndrome to ICU nurses, is sometimes missed if the patient's history of drinking is not known to the family or acknowledged in the admission interview. Even heavy coffee drinkers, who are dependent on large doses of caffeine, can show signs of withdrawal that contribute to agitation. By interviewing family members and reviewing the documented history and physical examination, the nurse may often determine the factors that are contributing to the patient's agitation.

Drug effects and hemodynamic and metabolic disturbances alter neurotransmission in the motor axis, reticular substance, basal ganglia, cerebellum, and motor cortex (Crippen & Ermakov, 1992; & Geary, 1994). The brain can no longer channel information to the cortical regions and interpret it on the basis of past memories. Instead, the input is mischanneled to lower regions of the brain—the basal ganglia, reticular formation, vestibular nuclei, and the extrapyramidal system. These regions respond with uncoordinated, nonpurposeful movements, tremors, musculoskeletal rigidity, and repetitive motion. Reactions may be highly emotional because of the dominance of lower, more primitive centers in the brain over higher regions, which would normally provide rational control.

If multisystem organ failure and persistent hypotension develop, the impact on the brain is profound. The prognosis is poor, and the patient may progress from delirium to coma (Geary, 1994).

Agitation, then, is a disturbance of brain function with behavioral and psychologic characteristics, which presents as globally impaired cognitive function, restlessness, rigidity and tremors, and alternating periods of hyperalertness and lethargy. Agitation is caused by impaired brain metabolism brought on by impaired delivery of oxygen and glucose to the brain or by metabolic disturbances, including drug toxicity or withdrawal. Psychologic stresses such as dyspnea, pain, and anxiety contribute to agitation, but they are not the primary cause of a reversible organic syndrome.

Because impaired brain metabolism is the primary etiology of agitation and confusion in critically ill patients, treatment is aimed at restoring normal brain function. After the assessment eliminates basic contributing factors such as hypoventilation, blocked airway, or faulty oxygen system, then appropriate steps should be taken to correct the underlying hemodynamic and metabolic disturbance. At the same time, pharmacologic agents are administered to restore equilibrium in neurotransmission and to suppress behaviors that are taxing the patient's reserves and jeopardizing care.

PHARMACOLOGIC MEASURES

The level and type of sedation used in the ICU have changed over the last two decades. In the past deep sedation in which the patient was completely detached from the environment was considered the ideal (Aitkenhead, 1989). Neuromuscular blocking agents were frequently administered (Shelly, 1994). The effects from these agents resulted in prolonged immobility and contributed to developing decubiti, congestive heart failure, pulmonary congestion, and aspiration of feeding material. By 1990 only 16% of ICUs used paralyzing agents (Shelly, 1994).

Today the goal of pharmacologic intervention is to relieve pain, anxiety, and other discomforts; to facilitate mechanical ventilation and other treatment modalities; and to provide amnesia for the more unpleasant aspects of critical illness. The preferred level of sedation is one in which the patient is asleep but easily roused and able to cooperate with care. This level also allows for patient mobility, including chair rest and turning side to side. The ideally sedated patient is calm, cooperative, and cognitively intact enough to broadly comprehend what is happening to and expected of the patient (Vitello et al., 1996).

While doing all that can be done to alleviate the source of the anxiety and discomfort, the RN may also administer one or more medications. If the discomfort is mild, the doses are similar to the conscious sedation protocols used in short-procedure units (e.g., endoscopy, surgery, or radiology). However, because of their abnormal brain chemistry, ICU patients frequently require larger doses of medication than are customarily administered to non-ICU patients (Barber, 1995; Crippen, 1994; & Harvey, 1996).

What is more, unless the patient is on a weaning mode, such as intermittent mandatory ventilation (IMV) or pressure support, mechanically ventilated patients are not in danger of respiratory arrest. Because anxiety and pain could impair synchrony with the ventilator, sedatives and analgesics improve oxygen exchange by slowing the respiratory rate, by allowing the patient to breathe with the ventilator, and by permitting the patient to cooperate with pulmonary toilet functions such as chest physiotherapy and coughing.

For several reasons the preferred route of administration in critical care is intravenous. First, oral medications are usually difficult to administer to the intubated patient, although some patients with tracheostomies are able to swallow pills, water, and even food. Absorption across the gastrointestinal (GI) tract is not always certain in these patients because of edematous bowel and decreased gastric motility. Also, as much as 90% of a sedative's bioavailability may be lost in passing through the GI tract and the liver (Aitkenhead, 1989; Luer, 1995).

The intravenous route offers improved efficacy and more accurate blood levels. It also provides a more rapid onset and allows for titration of administration, which is extremely useful for critically ill patients, whose condition may change abruptly. The intravenous route also avoids the local irritation to muscle produced by intramuscular or subcutaneous administration for several of the medications.

In deciding between on-request and regularly scheduled bolus administration (i.e., slow intravenous push), on-request sedation may lead to periods when the patient does not receive medication, and it is likely to produce even greater variations in blood levels than a regularly scheduled individual dose would. This gap in treatment can contribute to recurring agitation with negative consequences to the patient. Regularly scheduled sedatives and analgesics provide a steady state only after repeated doses. A bolus plus a continuous infusion of sedation that is supplemented by occasional miniboluses provides less variation in serum drug levels (i.e., a better steady state) than the bolus administration alone does.

There is currently no definitive evidence that continuous infusion of sedation yields a more effective relief of agitation than regularly scheduled bolus dosing. Bolus doses take four to five elimination half-lives to achieve a steady state (Aitkenhead, 1989; Riker, Gilles, & Cox, 1994). Advocates of the infusion method point out that bolus administration may not achieve a constant blood level of the medication for 24 hours or longer. The peak levels can cause oversedation and hemodynamic side effects. Trough levels can lead to new outbreaks of agitation, which puts the patient at risk of self-extubation (Shelly, 1994).

There is theoretic evidence that the patient can reach a steady state more quickly with a loading dose followed by a continuous infusion than with bolus dosing alone.

The infusion can be supplemented with miniboluses and the titration increased depending on the patient's level of sedation. Some clinicians believe it is possible to reach a steady state more quickly with the infusion/minibolus method (Aitkenhead, 1989; Luer, 1995).

The patient with a mild degree of anxiety or pain is given low to moderate doses of sedatives or analgesics, either in single doses or a loading dose and an infusion (Table 9-1). If discomfort is severe enough to cause agitation, higher doses are required (Table 9-2). The continuous infusion can be titrated up or down depending on the patient's level of sedation. If the patient shows signs of delirium, a neuroleptic may be added. It is important to keep in mind that, in addition to treating the patient's subjective state, the RN must continually seek the causes of the agitation and confusion and to treat those causes.

Frequently the combination of a benzodiazepine and opiate establish calm and comfort in the ICU patient (Crippen, 1994; Harvey, 1996; Luer, 1995). To treat confusion, a neuroleptic and a benzodiazepine are often combined. Because the drugs are synergistic, combination therapy allows for lower doses of each drug, thereby reducing risk for unwanted side effects. Results are better because anxiety, discomfort, and confusion are relieved.

Analgesics

Opiates are the mainstay of pain control in critical care. Their efficacy has been well established, and their side effects are known and in most cases controlled by adjusting the dose and rate of administration or by taking countermeasures such as intravenous fluids for transient hypotension. No other class of drugs has the efficacy of opiates.

Opiates bind to several discrete receptor sites in the brain and spinal cord. They decrease postsynaptic membrane response to excitatory transmitters such as norepinephrine and epinephrine (Barber, 1995), thereby decreasing the transmission of pain signals.

Despite the availability of opiates, as many as 50% of patients report that they received inadequate pain relief during their ICU stays, (Bizek, 1995; Carroll & Magruder, 1993; Harvey, 1996; Shelly, 1994). Past concerns about inducing addiction have proved unfounded. The persistence of apparent undertreatment of pain argues strongly for the use of pain assessment scales and the development of more accurate and comprehensive measuring devices.

Among the opiates meperidine is used less often than in the past because of its side effects (i.e., confusion, seizures, nausea, and vomiting) (Barber, 1995; Shapiro et al., 1995). Ketorlac tromethamine (Toradol), a nonopiate prostaglandin inhibitor, is becoming more popular for the relief of short-term pain, especially in the emergency department. However, Toradol does not have the potency or beneficial secondary effects of the opiates and is not approved for continuous intravenous infu-

TABLE 9-1 *Loading Dose, Infusion Rate, and Titration for Low to Moderate Signs/Symptoms of Anxiety and Discomfort**

DRUG	LOAD	INFUSE	TITRATE
Morphine	1-5 mg	1-5 mg/hr	1 mg
Fentanyl	50-100 μg	50-250 μg/hr	50 μg
Diazepam	2-5 mg	2-5 mg/hr	2 mg
Lorazepam	1-2 mg	1-4 mg/hr	1 mg
Midazolam	0.5-1.5 mg	1-5 mg/hr	0.5 mg
Propofol	50-150 mg	50-150 mg/hr	50 mg
Haloperidol	2-10 mg	2-10 mg/hr†	1-2 mg

*Patient weighs 70 kg.
†If no improvement in patient condition after 20 to 30 minutes, double dose. Check intravenous infusion over time.
NOTE: Literature supports administration of haloperidol in slowly increasing doses.

TABLE 9-2 *Loading Dose, Infusion Rate, and Titration for Moderate to Severe Signs/Symptoms of Anxiety and Discomfort**

DRUG	LOAD	INFUSE	TITRATE
Morphine	5-15 mg	5-10 mg/hr	2 mg
Fentanyl	100-200 μg	100 μg	75-1200 μg
Diazepam	5-10 mg	5-10 mg/hr	3-5 mg
Lorazepam	2-10 mg	2-10 mg/hr	2 mg
Midazolam	1.5-3 mg	5-7 mg	1 mg
Propofol	150-300 mg	150-300 mg/hr	75-100 mg
Haloperidol	10-100 mg	10-50 mg/hr†	5 mg

*Patient weighs 70 kg.
†If no improvement in patient condition after 20 to 30 minutes, double dose. Check intravenous infusion over time.
NOTE: Literature supports administration of haloperidol in slowly increasing doses.

sion. Morphine and fentanyl are currently the most commonly prescribed opiates in critical care.

Morphine

Morphine is a pure opiate agonist that binds to opiate receptor sites in the central and peripheral nervous system. Morphine blocks the transmission and perception of pain. Morphine is given intravenously to avoid local irritation of intramuscular or subcutaneous injections. Because it is not lipophilic, morphine has a slower onset than fentanyl. Once a therapeutic blood level has been established, it provides relief for 2 to 4 hours.

Morphine's actions can affect the cardiac, pulmonary, GI, and neurohormonal systems. It is known to stimulate histamine release, which causes hypotension because of peripheral vasodilation. The decreased preload lowers filling pressures in the right side of the heart. Hypotension is more common and more pronounced in patients with hypovolemia or decreased left ventricular function. Patients with a reduced peripheral vasoconstrictive response, which may be the result of paralysis, diabetic neuropathy, or administration of α-blocking medication, are vulnerable to opiate-induced hypotension. These patients should receive lower doses of morphine that are administered slowly.

An opiate's undesirable effects on the cardiovascular system are particularly advantageous for the pulmonary system in a mechanically ventilated patient. The reduced preload decreases congestion in the pulmonary capillary bed, increasing pulmonary compliance. This enhances alveolar expansion and gas exchange, a phenomenon that is often seen when administering morphine intravenously to patients with flash pulmonary edema. Symptoms are reduced quickly and dramatically, peak airway pressures are lowered, and chest x-ray films demonstrate improvement in pulmonary congestion.

Opiates decrease gastric motility, leading to constipation and a potential small bowel ileus. Gastric emptying may be slowed; nausea and vomiting create a risk for aspiration pneumonia, even with an inflated cuff balloon. Patients receiving enteral support should be assessed frequently (i.e., every 2 to 4 hours) for abdominal distention and residual gastric feeding. The frequency, amount, and quality of bowel movements should be documented so that constipation can be identified and treated early.

There is laboratory evidence that morphine inhibits the immune response in mice. This finding has not been proved in human subjects, but the possibility of impairing resistance to infection should be kept in mind (Luer, 1995).

With good pain relief the patient is able to relax, allowing for easier chest excursion, improving thoracic compliance. The patient is able to cooperate with suctioning and chest physiotherapy. The actions, advantages, disadvantages, and unwanted side effects of morphine are summarized in Table 9-3.

By diluting 10 mg of morphine in 10 ml of sterile water, the drug can be administered in 1 ml doses every 5 to 10 minutes until the patient is comfortable. A slow administration minimizes cardiac side effects.

On administration of intravenous opiates, there is a rapid rise in blood levels. The serum level drops off as the drug diffuses into the third space, soft tissue, and bone marrow. A second dose yields a higher serum drug level because the medication has already become bound to receptor sites and been distributed throughout the body. A higher serum level results in a higher rate of elimination, assuming a normal liver and renal function.

TABLE 9-3 *Summary of Medications Used in Treatment of Agitation and Delirium*

MEDICATION	ACTIONS/ADVANTAGES	SIDE EFFECTS/DISADVANTAGES
Fentanyl	Crosses blood-brain barrier more readily than morphine sulfate More rapid onset when given in low to moderate dose Produces less hypotension than morphine sulfate	Respiratory depression Hypotension May cause glottic rigidity if given rapidly, complicating intubation May cause sleep deprivation
Ketorlac	Sustained pain relief Does not cause hypotension	Less effective than opiates
Diazepam	Rapid onset Effective anxiolysis Easily and quickly reversed Good musculoskeletal relaxation	Irritates small veins Precipitates in intravenous lines and solutions Hypotension Active metabolite extends elimination half-life Respiratory depressant
Lorazepam	Rapid onset Effective anxiolysis No active metabolites Inexpensive	Precipitates in intravenous lines and solution Solution must be changed every 12 hours Respiratory depression Hypotension Slower onset than midazolam
Midazolam	Rapid onset Effective anxiolysis Not irritating to veins Does not precipitate in solution	Respiratory depression Hypotension Expensive Has active metabolite
Propofol	Rapid onset Effective sedation Rapid clearance shortens wake-up time Effective for patient with opiate tolerance/addiction	Hypotension Respiratory depression Potential for bacterial contamination No reversing agent available
Haloperidol	Blocks dopamine at postsynaptic receptor sites Relieves confusion, tremors	Extramyramidal symptoms Prolongs Q-T interval May induce torsades des pointes May cause neuroleptic malignant syndrome Exacerbates symptoms of Parkinson's disease
Clonidine	Inhibits norepinephrine release centrally Reduces anxiety, restlessness Synergy allows lower doses of opiates and benzodiazepines	Hypotension Bradycardia, conduction blocks
Morphine	Quickly reversed Short half-life makes it rapidly titratable	May cause hypotension due to decreased preload (vasodilation) Decreases gastric motility and may induce ileus or vomiting May cause histamine release and decreased bronchoconstriction

If the patient receives opiates for more than 5 days, the elimination half-life may be extended (Table 9-4). This prolongation of half-life may be due to liver failure, which metabolizes the opiate, or renal failure, which excretes the active metabolite. The exact mechanisms that effect drug elimination in the critically ill patient are not known.

Because morphine is not lipophilic, it is relatively slow to cross the liporich blood-brain barrier. The drug becomes distributed in the third space and internal organs and enters bone marrow. It is metabolized by the liver and excreted by the kidneys and in bile salts.

The distribution of opiates is altered as a result of fluid retention, a common problem in critically ill patients. Mechanical ventilation causes a decrease in blood return to the heart, which promotes increased antidiuretic hormone (ADH) production and a resultant sodium and water retention. Because opiates must diffuse into a relatively large extracellular volume, the patient may require higher doses than those given for the ideal weight.

If microcirculation is compromised, as in shock states, ischemic processes, or sepsis, opiates may be sequestered in poorly perfused tissue for prolonged periods of time. This may lead to reabsorption and resedation several hours or even days after opiates have been discontinued.

The abnormal brain function of agitated, critically ill patients further contributes to the need for higher doses of opiates. The excessive production of norepinephrine antagonizes the effects of opiates. Dopamine surges induce restlessness, sleeplessness, and musculoskeletal rigidity. These symptoms may not resolve unless relatively high doses of opiates are administered.

TABLE 9-4 *Normal and Extended Elimination Half-Lives of Sedating Agents Used in ICU*

DRUG	NON-ICU PATIENT HALF-LIFE (hr)	ICU PATIENT HALF-LIFE (hr)	ACTIVE METABOLITE AND ITS HALF-LIFE (hr)
Morphine	1.5-4	5.9-13	M6G
Fentanyl	2-5	9-16	None
Diazepam	24-36	36-72	N-desmethyl diazepam
Lorazepam	15	No available data	None
Midazolam	1-4	5-26	
Propofol	1.5-3	24-30	None
Haloperidol	10-40	40-100	None
Flumazenil	0.6-1.3	Unknown	
Naloxone	0.5-1	0.5-1.3	

An initial dose of morphine, 2 to 10 mg given by slow intravenous injection, is given for mild to moderate pain; 10 to 15 mg is given for moderate to severe pain. Cardiac parameters must be closely monitored. The loading dose may be followed by an infusion of 2 to 10 mg/hr, with additional small boluses if pain recurs. The dose is titrated until the patient is comfortable, provided cardiac parameters are within acceptable limits.

Morphine has the active metabolite M6G, which can remain in the serum for several hours. Even when the parent drug, morphine, is broken down by the liver and excreted, the psychoactive metabolite can significantly extend the wake-up time.

Opiates given to the ICU patient have been shown to undergo an unusually prolonged elimination half-life (Aitkenhead, 1989; & Harvey, 1996). The change in the drug's pharmacokinetics has been attributed to impaired liver or renal function, low serum albumin levels, and sequestration of active metabolites in poorly perfused tissue. Shock states may dramatically increase elimination times. The exact mechanism, or mechanisms, is not well understood.

Prolonged elimination times can produce abnormally high serum drug levels. If the dose is not titrated downward, oversedation and unwanted side effects can occur. These can be avoided by careful patient assessment, by the use of a sedation scale, and by considering the patient's age and liver and renal function. Any patient who is hypotensive or who receives a continuous morphine infusion should be assessed frequently (e.g., hourly neurologic assessment) for increased opiate effects.

Fentanyl

Fentanyl is an opiate agonist that is becoming increasingly popular in the ICU because of its rapid onset. A highly lipophilic drug, fentanyl readily crosses the blood-brain barrier and binds with receptor sites in the brain and spinal cord.

Like morphine, fentanyl can cause hypotension and a decreased respiratory rate as a result of lowered sensitivity to carbon dioxide receptors in the brain. Constipation, nausea, and vomiting and decreased gastric emptying may also occur. A large loading dose may induce glottic rigidity, complicating intubation. If fentanyl is chosen before intubation for its rapid onset, it should be given in low to moderate amounts.

Even with its rapid onset, fentanyl has a longer elimination half-life than morphine does. This longer half-life is more likely to occur in patients who have received fentanyl infusions for more than 3 to 5 days (Luer, 1995; Wheeler, 1993) or who have liver or renal failure. Its lipophilicity causes fentanyl to be stored in fatty tissue, from which it is slowly released into the blood. This may lead to oversedation after several days of administration or to resedation after the medication is discontinued (Crippen & Ermakov, 1992). Careful titration and monitoring with a sedation scale, along with attention to factors that extend the drug's efficacy, will prevent excessive accumulation in the body.

Because of its potential for slow elimination, fentanyl infusions should be stopped if the patient shows signs of oversedation or hypotension. The gradual drop-off of drug levels after bolus and intravenous infusions suggests that merely lowering the infusion rate will not produce a rapid decline in blood levels because the infusion continues to administer the drug. Stopping the opiate until the unwanted side effects have resolved and restarting at a lower rate produce a more rapid resolution of the problem. Weaning must be done more slowly than in patients receiving short-term analgesia or sedation.

For low to moderate discomfort, 50 to 100 µg is administered intravenously over 1 to 2 minutes. This may be followed by an infusion of 50 to 100 µg/hr. If the patient remains uncomfortable and hemodynamic parameters are within acceptable limits, a minibolus of 50 µg is given, after which the infusion may be increased by 50 µg/hr. This regimen is repeated until the patient is comfortable. Fentanyl will improve synchrony with the ventilator, diminish pulmonary congestion, and improve pulmonary parameters such as peak airway pressure.

Anxiolytics and Hypnotics

The benzodiazepines are the agents most commonly used in the ICU to relieve anxiety, restore normal sleep, provide amnesia, and relax skeletal muscles. No other class of medications provides the efficacy and low risk of complications as the benzodiazepines. They are often used concomitantly with opiates or neuroleptics, creating a synergy that affords improved comfort and allows for lower doses of each agent.

These agents appear to bind with benzodiazepine receptor sites in the central nervous system (CNS), where they potentate or mimic the inhibitory neurotransmitter GABA (Crippen, 1994) and glycine (Barber, 1995). They reduce anxiety, produce dose-dependant amnesia, and relax skeletal muscles. The three most commonly administered benzodiazepines in the ICU include diazepam, lorazepam, and midazolam.

Diazepam

Diazepam (Valium) was the most commonly prescribed intravenous benzodiazepine in the 1980s (Shelly, 1994). It is a long-acting sedative that has become less frequently used in the ICU because of its prolonged duration and undesirable side effects. Diazepam has the advantage of a rapid onset of 1 to 5 minutes because of its high lipid solubility. It provides effective relief of anxiety and muscle rigidity and is often effective for acute cessation of seizures. Diazepam is metabolized by the liver and excreted by the kidneys.

For mild to moderate agitation, diazepam is given slowly in a 2 to 5 mg dose. For moderate to severe agitation, a 5 to 10 mg dose may be used. Infusion rates of 2 to 10 mg/hr are common. If diazepam alone does not relieve the patient's agitation, in combination with an opiate it is very effective. When combination therapy is used, smaller doses of each medication are indicated to prevent excessive side effects.

Diazepam may produce respiratory depression by suppressing carbon dioxide sensitivity in the brain, and it may cause hypotension because of peripheral vascular dilatation. Its major disadvantage is its prolonged effect. This is due in part to diazepam's long elimination half-life of 24 to 72 hours. Its active metabolite, *N*-desmethyl diazepam, has an elimination half-life of up to 96 hours. Even when the parent drug, diazepam, has been metabolized in the liver, the metabolite's CNS-depressing effects continue.

Phlebitis in a peripheral vein may result from the propylene glycol used as the vehicle for intravenous diazepam. Diazepam also easily precipitates out in normal saline solution or Ringer's lactate solution. For slow intravenous administration it should be mixed in sterile water in a 1:1 or 1:2 dilution and given slowly over 1 to 2 minutes. This will minimize local irritation and excessive sedation or hypotension.

When mixed in a solution for continuous administration, diazepam easily precipitates. The solution must be checked frequently for signs of precipitation and discarded if such signs are visible.

Lorazepam

Lorazepam is an intermediate-acting sedative with a slower onset than diazepam or midazolam. Because it does not have an active metabolite, its sedating effects are removed as it is metabolized by the liver, and it does not depend on renal function to excrete active metabolites, as is the case with diazepam and midazolam.

A 1 to 2 mg intravenous dose is administered to the patient with mild to moderate agitation. This may be followed by regularly scheduled intravenous boluses or by a continuous infusion of 1 to 2 mg/hr. The more severely agitated patient may require 2 to 4 mg. As with all benzodiazepines, patients with a history of benzodiazepine use, such as alprazolam (Xanax), require higher doses of this sedative or combination with an opiate or propofol.

Lorazepam's disadvantages are that it, like diazepam, precipitates easily. For this reason, it should be mixed in a glass bottle, and the bottle and tubing should be changed every 12 hours. As with any benzodiazepine, lorazepam may cause respiratory depression or hypotension.

Midazolam

Midazolam is a short-acting benzodiazepine with good sedating and amnesic properties. A water-soluble preparation, midazolam does not irritate peripheral veins, nor does it precipitate in solutions or intravenous lines. It has a rapid onset, and when used for fewer than 3 to 5 days, has an elimination half-life of 2 to 4 hours. However, after long-term use midazolam's elimination half-life may be extended to 5 to 26 hours. This occurs when the drug is sequestered in poorly perfused fatty tissue, its metabolism is slowed due to liver failure, or its elimination is diminished because of renal failure. These conditions cause midazolam to act more like an intermediate-acting rather than a short-acting drug in critically ill patients. Its active metabolite has an elimination half-life of 1 hour.

An intravenous dose of 0.5 to 1.5 mg is given over 1 minute. Patients more than 65 years old or with chronic obstructive pulmonary disease (COPD) are initially given the lowest dose to avoid respiratory depression. Peak effect occurs in 2 to 3 minutes. Repeat doses of 0.5 mg may be given after 4 to 5 minutes until the patient is adequately sedated. Patients receiving opiates should be given one third to one fifth the normal dose of midazolam. Hypotension and respiratory depression are possible side effects.

Propofol

Propofol (Diprivan), a nonbenzodiazepine, nonopiate anesthetic, is relatively new to critical care sedation. Used for more than 8 years in the operating room as an anesthetic, propofol in lower doses provides excellent conscious sedation in the ICU for the mechanically ventilated patient. As critical care nurses become familiar with its actions and titration, propofol is coming into wider use.

Propofol has a very rapid onset and rapid termination. The patient does not receive a loading dose, as is common with opiates and benzodiazepines. Some anesthesiologists administer a very small test dose to be sure there is no allergic reaction. Because it can be irritating to the vein, the infusion is initiated slowly and gradually increased as the patient becomes somnolent.

An infusion of 50 to 150 mg/hr provides light to moderate sedation in a 70 kg adult. The infusion may be increased by 50 mg up to a dose of 300 mg/hr (Stuart Pharmaceuticals, 1993). The most common side effect is hypotension from peripheral vasodilation, which is more likely in the patient who is hypovolemic or elderly or who has decreased left ventricular function.

The normal elimination half-life is 4 to 9 hours, but this does not correlate with the normal wake-up time, which is 10 to 30 minutes. As with opiates and benzodiazepines, the elimination half-life in the critically ill patient has been found to extend to 24 to 30 hours for the same reasons as the other sedating drugs. This may extend wake-up times, although clinical experience has not confirmed this.

Propofol is suspended in a 10% lipid solution, which may have unwanted side effects. When lipids are metabolized they break down to carbon dioxide and water. Elevations of arterial carbon dioxide of 5% to 10% have been documented in patients with COPD who have received propofol. Elevated serum triglyceride and glucose levels have been found in patients with a restricted ability to metabolize fat. Patients receiving intravenous hyperalimentation should have their caloric intakes adjusted if they are to receive long-term propofol infusions.

The most serious unwanted side effect reported in the literature is bacteremia. There have been documented cases of patients having bacterial infection because of contamination of the propofol solute. This danger can be prevented with the use of scrupulous aseptic technique when handling the medication. Some hospital protocols require that the intravenous solution containing propofol and the tubing be changed every 12 hours to prevent contamination. The site must be carefully checked for signs of local infection, and any sign of bacterial colonization warrants discontinuing the drug and changing the intravenous site.

Propofol is classified as an aphrodisiac. It is known to cause vivid sexual dreams. Patients and families should be cautioned before propofol sedation is initiated that the patient may experience sexual dreams and they are not to confuse them with real experience. Currently there is no reversal agent for this drug.

Neuroleptics and Sympathetic Inhibiting Agents

Delirium in the critically ill patient is caused by a reversible organic syndrome caused by impaired brain metabolism. Abnormal neurotransmission results in loss of cognitive function, restlessness and tremulousness, uncontrolled motor activity, and musculoskeletal rigidity. This syndrome is often a sign that one or more organ systems are deteriorating and should elicit an immediate assessment of all patient parameters. These include vital signs, arterial oxygen, pH and carbon dioxide levels, liver and renal function, and glucose levels. All medications should be reviewed for possible toxicity, and the patient's history of medication or drug abuse should be scrutinized.

Although treatment of the underlying causes of delirium is the primary focus of care, the confusional state may continue for hours or even days. In these cases medications are administered to restore a more normal neurotransmission.

Chlorpromazine hydrochloride (Thorazine) was one of the early antipsychotic medications. Its use has been curtailed by unwanted side effects, including leukopenia, extrapyramidal symptoms, electrocardiographic changes, including widened QRS and QT intervals, and constipation.

Chlorpromazine use has been generally replaced by haloperidol, which has fewer unwanted side effects and provides better relief of symptoms.

Haloperidol

Haloperidol (Haldol) is the drug of choice for delirium in the ICU. Extensive experiences documented in more than 700 articles demonstrate haloperidol's efficacy and low incidence of unwanted side effects. It has no analgesic or sedating properties, but because it relieves confusion it may help the patient achieve a calm state when confusion is frightening.

Haloperidol acts by blocking surges of dopamine from several regions of the brain, including the limbic system. By suppressing the effects of this neurotransmitter, haloperidol relieves restlessness, tremors, and uncontrolled muscle movements, as well as disorientation. It helps restore organized thinking, which enables the patient to better comprehend what is happening.

Side effects of haloperidol include extrapyramidal symptoms, laryngospasm, and bronchospasm. Rarely, a neuromalignant syndrome has been reported. Its symptoms include high fever, tachycardia, hypotension, muscle stiffness, diaphoresis, and autonomic instability. The drug must be discontinued immediately if these signs occur, and interventions must be aimed at specific abnormalities. Fever is corrected, fluid resuscitation, cooling therapies, and dopamine agonist (amantadine hydrochloride) may be used.

The QT interval should be measured every shift and documented because haloperidol has been associated with widening a QT and torsades des pointes, a potentially fatal arrhythmia. If a prolonged QT interval develops, the haloperidol should be stopped, the physician notified, and all serum electrolyte levels checked. Low serum potassium and magnesium have been associated with increased risk of torasades des pointes. Serum levels should be brought to a high normal level in the face of this electrocardiographic change.

Haloperidol is contraindicated for patients with a history of Parkinson's disease, a disease of decreased dopamine production in the brain. Because haloperidol blocks dopamine, it can worsen signs and symptoms of this disease.

Intravenous administration is the most effective route. The recommended dose is 2 to 10 mg intravenously. If symptoms are not improved in 20 to 30 minutes, the dose can be doubled. If symptoms are not improved in 30 minutes, the dose can be doubled again. This regimen is continued until the patient improves, or until the dose exceeds hospital protocols.

If haloperidol alone does not resolve signs of delirium, combination with a benzodiazepine has been shown to be efficacious. As with any combination, the amount of each medication should be reduced because of the synergy. Adding a benzodiazepine also reduces the incidence of side effects from haloperidol.

Clonidine

Clonidine is an α-adrenergic agonist that inhibits the release of norepinephrine from central and peripheral presynaptic junctions by a negative feedback mechanism (Crippen & Ermakov, 1992). Excessive production of catecholamines is thought to be linked to ICU delirium, especially to hyperalertness, sleep intolerance, and tremulousness. By blocking this potent neurotransmitter, clonidine reduces signs and symptoms of agitation.

Administration of opiates for more than 5 days has been implicated with excessive norepinephrine release (Farrell, 1994; & Kosten & McCance, 1996). Clonidine is especially helpful for these patients. It enables the use of lower doses of opiates to achieve comfort, thereby reducing the risk of hypotension or respiratory depression. Clonidine is also thought to have analgesic properties, although the mechanism of action is not known (Crippen & Ermakov, 1992).

Clonidine also acts synergistically with benzodiazepines and with haloperidol. It helps to relieve confusion and agitation and allows for lower doses of both drugs.

The loading dose is 0.1 to 1.0 mg orally twice daily, depending on the severity of symptoms. A transdermal patch releasing 0.1 to 0.3 mg/hr can be added after the loading dose is given orally. An intravenous preparation has been used in Europe and is currently undergoing clinical trials in the United States. When it is approved, intravenous clonidine is likely to become an important adjunct to treatment for agitation in the ICU.

Combination Therapy

Many clinicians obtain improved effects by combining opiates, benzodiazepines, neuroleptics, and propofol in varying combinations. The choice of agents depends on the specific disorder being treated and on how well the patient tolerates each class of medication. If raising the dose of a single medication does not resolve the patient's discomfort or agitation, adding a second drug often yields improved results.

Each class of drugs works synergistically with the others. For this reason it is important to lower the dose of each one. Continuous infusions may be run concomitantly. Bolus administrations may be alternated, so that the patient receives a medication frequently.

An example of a combination therapy is lorazepam 4 mg intravenously every 4 hours around the clock and haloperidol 10 mg intravenously every 4 hours to alternate with lorazepam. With this regimen the patient receives a sedating or calming medication every 2 hours.

Propofol can be combined with opiates. The propofol infusion is given in a lower infusion rate because the hypotensive effects can be magnified by the combined drug effects.

Combination therapy is particularly advantageous in preventing tolerance and when weaning a patient. There are reports that after 5 to 7 days of intravenous sedation prolonged elimination half-lives of the drug develop.

Tolerance and Extended Elimination Half-Lives

Tolerance is the phenomenon of requiring progressively higher doses of a medication to obtain the same results. It is why a heroin addict requires increasing amounts of an opiate to experience positive effects. In the ICU patients who have no history of drug addiction may begin to show signs of opiate tolerance in 5 to 7 days. They may report inadequate pain relief after receiving the previously effective dose.

This tolerance results from the body's natural tendency to respond to a continuous CNS-depressing effect. Opiates and benzodiazepines dull sensation. After receiving repeated doses, the body produces increasing amounts of excitatory neurotransmitters. In response to chronic opiate use, the brain produces large amounts of norepinephrine in the locus coereleus. The brain also increases the sensitivity of nore-pinephrine receptors, almost as if it were trying to rouse itself from a forced slumber.

The stimulatory effects of excitatory transmitters counteract the sedating effects of opiates and benzodiazepines. The RN is forced to administer higher doses of medication to achieve a satisfactory level of comfort for the patient.

One way to avoid or reduce tolerance is to use combination drug therapy. Benzodiazepines, which reduce the anxiety that contributes to pain, work synergistically with opiates, allowing for lower dosing of the analgesic. This combination slows the development of opiate tolerance.

For patients who require high doses of benzodiazepines, the addition of haloperidol allows better control of agitation and confusion, as well as lowering dose of the sedative (Luer, 1995).

Several theories have been brought forth to explain the extended half-life of opiates and sedatives. Liver failure slows the metabolism of these medications and plays an important role. Renal insufficiency or failure impair elimination of the active metabolites, which contributes to the drugs' sedating properties. With low serum albumin levels, a common finding in the ICU patient, analgesics and sedatives are less able to bind to protein for transport to the brain.

Compromised microcirculation plays a role in prolonging drug half-lives. Poorly perfused tissues store drugs for prolonged periods. After the serum level has dropped, stores of the drug slowly diffuse into the bloodstream and are transported to the brain and spinal cord, causing resedation and unwanted side effects. A sedation scale may also be continued for 24 to 48 hours after a sedative is discontinued as a way to monitor the patient's level of consciousness and comfort.

NONPHARMACOLOGIC MEASURES

Direct interventions to relieve the patient's discomfort are an essential part of nursing care. The goal is to correct the condition that is causing the discomfort and to initiate interventions that promote comfort and a sense of well-being.

Because dyspnea and pain are common problems in the ventilated patient, every effort is made to assess for the causes. The dyspneic patient is examined for bilateral breath sounds, signs of bronchial constriction, accumulation of secretions, and proper endotracheal tube placement. Suctioning is done to remove secretions and to assess for changes in pulmonary flora and for the presence of blood or frothy sputum, suggesting pulmonary emboli or edema, respectively.

Ventilatory parameters are evaluated for changes in the patient's condition. Rising peak airway pressures may signify pneumothorax, airway plugging, or decreased lung compliance as a result of adult respiratory distress syndrome (ARDS). Decreased expiratory volumes suggest an air leak, which may be caused by improper tube placement, inadequate seal by the balloon, or breaks or loose connections in the tubing, caps, or nebulizer. Increased minute ventilation is a nonspecific sign that the patient is not adequately oxygenating the tissues. It does not pinpoint the cause as pulmonary organ failure but directs attention to impaired gas exchange or delivery. An internal failure of the ventilator itself must also be considered.

If the endotracheal tube is not in the trachea, as evidenced by patient vocalization and air movement from the nose and mouth during mechanically assisted inspiration, the tube should be removed. The patient is manually ventilated with 100% oxygen and an anesthesia provider is paged STAT. Intubation equipment and extra sedation is brought to the bedside in preparation for reintubation. The patient's oxygen saturation, color, and vital signs are closely observed.

Pain can originate from sources that are sometimes overlooked. Because the patient has difficulty communicating information, it may be difficult to ascertain the precise location and type of pain. A patient who points to the upper abdomen or lower chest may be indicating chest pain, abdominal pain, inferior pleuritic pain, pancreatic, or gall bladder pain. Often only a complete physical assessment and thorough review of laboratory values will reveal the probable source of the discomfort.

Other physical discomforts afflicting the patient may be nausea and the urge to vomit, which can be terrifying to the intubated patient who cannot easily turn and expectorate gastric material. An itch that cannot be scratched, a sensation of cold or fever, a need to urinate or defecate, or the desire to change position and relieve stiffened joints may be extremely disquieting to the patient. The patient's inability to communicate these needs can further heighten the discomfort and lead to agitation.

Anxiety arises from many sources that are not always apparent. Identifying the source often requires effort and imagination. Patients are often extremely troubled by the fear of painful procedures, the loss of control over activities of daily living, and the dependence on strangers to provide necessities of life. These necessities include a constant supply of oxygen, nutrition, fluids, and the elimination of urine and feces, activities of daily living that the healthy individual may take for granted. The patient's abrupt change from independent to dependent person can be deeply disturbing to the patient and to the family.

Critical illness presents a family with a major crisis. Issues related to employment and income, responsibility and leadership in the family, and other personal issues stress the patient. Frequently, the patient is separated from significant others at a time when the patient has a heightened need for their emotional support. Spouses of many years may find forced separation frightening or depressing.

Some ICUs have introduced liberal visiting hours. Others maintain strict limits on the number of visitors allowed and the length of the visit. There is a growing trend to allow more liberal visitations as hospitals recognize the impact of isolation on the critically ill patient, but practices vary widely among institutions and at times even among critical care units within an institution.

Communication for the mechanically ventilated patient is difficult. In addition, it is sometimes complicated by a language barrier. Hospitals may maintain a list of bilingual employees to provide translators who assist in taking a history and providing information and reassurance to the patient and family.

Cards with phrases and translations can help relieve a patient's anxiety. Basic needs are expressed, and broad information about the patient's prognosis, probable length of stay, and the need for further diagnostic tests and treatments can be conveyed to the patient.

Confusion can cause a patient much anxiety, especially if hallucinations or delusions accompany it. The RN must make every effort to reorient the patient while at the same time validating the patient's feelings. Phrases such as, "I'm sure you feel frightened, Mr. Smith. I would feel the same way, but I can assure you that you are in a hospital, I am your nurse, and we are treating you for pneumonia. Do you understand?" support the patient's emotions while redirecting the patient toward a more realistic appraisal of reality.

Many institutions try to soften the harsh environment with soft lighting, restful music, and pleasant interior designs. Attempts to restore a normal sleep cycle can be hampered by excessive auditory and tactile stimuli. Efforts should be taken to prevent false alarms (e.g., secure electrocardiograph electrode placement) and unnecessary noise.

Orientation to time and place may be enhanced by the use of large clocks and calendars and by reading highlights from a daily newspaper, including the weather report. Pictures from home not only help the patient recall loved ones but remind caregivers of the patient's identity before becoming critically ill, nonverbal because of the endotracheal tube, and possibly disoriented.

SEDATION SCALE AND OTHERS MEASURES OF SEDATION

In the past decade the use of sedation scales has increased for the patient receiving intravenous sedation. Sedation scales serve two basic functions: (1) they measure the patient's subjective state (e.g., pain, anxiety, confusion, or other discomforts) and (2) they measure the objective behaviors that usually accompany internal tension (e.g., restlessness, hyperreflexia, inability to sleep, tremulousness, and musculoskeletal rigidity).

Sedation scales also provide a means to define the goal, which is the desired level of sedation. This measures the efficacy of treatment and tells the practitioner whether the interventions have been successful. Sedation scales may assist the practitioner avoid undersedation or oversedation. Studies have shown that by using a sedation scale the RN is able to establish the desired sedation level more quickly and safely (Harvey, 1996).

One widely used sedation scale in the ICU setting is the Ramsay scale. It is a simple six-point sedation score that focuses on the agitated patient requiring sedation. The Ramsay scale measures three levels of waking and three levels of sleep (Table 9-

5) showing different levels of variable responses to loud noise, verbal communication, and glabellar tapping. When used as a guide for sedating the patient, the physician orders medication to be given to achieve a specific Ramsay score. The medication may be ordered to be given as needed, in which case the RN administers medication until the desired level of sedation is reached. Or the medication dose may be variable, within preprescribed limits, which the RN adjusts in line with the patient's level of agitation and discomfort.

The preferred depth of sedation has changed considerably in the last 15 years. In the past a deep level of sleep, which would today be measured as a 5 or 6 on the Ramsay scale, was frequently the goal. Today, most practitioners aim for a lighter level of sedation, usually a Ramsay score of 2 or 3. Patients with severe pulmonary disease who require high levels of positive end-expiratory pressure or experience persistent, marked degrees of dyspnea often require a deeper level of sedation. The higher doses promote muscle relaxation and improve pulmonary compliance.

One major limitation of the Ramsay scale is that is was never validated by objective measures (Hansen-Flaschen, Cowen, & Polomano, 1994; Harper, 1994). There is ambiguity and overlap in some of the categories. For example, a patient who is intermittently sleeping and who awakens to verbal stimuli (level 4) may be anxious and restless (level 1). Also, different raters who simultaneously observe the same patient have been known to assign different Ramsay scores to the patient.

Other limitations of the Ramsay scale include the lack of focus on the specific type of discomfort causing the agitation or confusion. Because this scale does not identify levels of pain, dyspnea, or anxiety, it is difficult to use the score to evaluate the efficacy of specific treatments.

Some institutions have adopted an algorithm approach to managing the uncomfortable patient. This method begins by assessing for anxiety, pain, dyspnea, or delirium. The nurse then identifies probable causes for each problem. The algorithm then suggests treatments specific to each type of problem. Although the algorithm does not measure level of sedation as such, it does address the need to identify specific problems that produce agitation or confusion.

Luer (1995) developed an eight-point scale that addresses specific sources of agitation in the mechanically ventilated patient (see Table 9-5). The categories include problems such as asynchrony with the ventilator, decreased oxygen saturation, and increased heart rate. The score ranges include the following: score 1, the combative patient who interferes with care and has a severe potential for self-harm; score 2, the anxious, agitated, or fearful patient who is moderately at risk; score 3, the restless patient with a mild potential for harm; score 4, the awake, calm, cooperative patient; score 5, the sleeping but arousable patient; score 6, the patient who is difficult to arouse by verbal stimuli; score 7, the minimally responsive patient; and score 8, the unresponsive patient.

Luer's categories include recommendations for the frequency of drug administration. For example, the combative patient receives a sedative every 30 minutes;

TABLE 9-5 Comparison of Different Sedation Scales

PATIENT CONDITION	FREQUENCY OF ASSESSMENT/MEDICATION	SCORE
RAMSAY SCALE		
Level 1 Patient awake, anxious and agitated or restless (or both)		
Level 2 Patient awake, cooperative, oriented, and tranquil		
Level 3 Patient awake; responds to commands only		
Level 4 Patient asleep; brisk response to light glabellar tap or loud auditory stimulus		
Level 5 Patient asleep; sluggish response to light glabellar tap or loud auditory stimulus		
Level 6 Patient asleep; no response to light glabellar tap or loud auditory stimulus		
LUER SCALE (ABRIDGED)		
Combative; interferes with care; severe potential for self-harm	Every 30 minutes Repeat loading dose	1
Anxious, agitated, fearful/ moderate potential for self-harm	Every hour Repeat loading dose	2
Restless; mild potential for self-harm/ objective parameter (e.g., asynchronous breathing, low oxygen saturation)	Every 2 hours Give 50% loading dose	3
Awake, calm, and cooperative; follows commands	Every 4 hours Maintain infusion; consider titrating down after 24 hours	4
Asleep but arousable	Every 4 hours Decrease infusion 0.5 mg	5
Difficult to arouse by verbal stimuli	Every hour	6
Minimal or no response to tactile stimuli	Every hour; decrease infusion 1 mg; notify physician	7
No response to painful stimuli	Call physician, stop infusion	8
SHELLY SCALE		
Eyes open		
Spontaneously		4
To speech		3
To pain		2
None		1
Response to nursing procedures		
Obeys commands		4
Purposeful movements		3
Nonpurposeful movement		2
None		1

TABLE 9-5 *Comparison of Different Sedation Scales—cont'd*	
PATIENT CONDITION	SCORE
Cough	
Spontaneous, strong	4
Spontaneous, weak	3
On suction only	2
None	1
Respirations	
Extubated	5
Spontaneous, intubated	4
IMV-triggered respiration	3
Respiration against ventilator	2
No respiratory effort	1

the less agitated, an hourly sedation; the restless patient, a sedative every 2 hours; and so on. For the unresponsive patient, the sedation is stopped and the physician notified.

The eight-point scale offers a more comprehensive neurologic assessment than the Ramsay scale does. It also suggests problem-oriented interventions, somewhat like the algorithm. Luer's scale appears to have some advantages over the others and warrants further clinical study.

A somewhat different approach taken by Shelly identifies four problems that can cause agitation and impair mechanical ventilation. The four problems identified include level of consciousness, ability to cooperate with nursing procedures, ability to assist with pulmonary toilet, and the degree of ventilatory support required (see Table 9-5). This scale is a useful way to categorize problems because it is goal-directed. Improvement in patient outcomes can be discerned by noting specific scores and the patient's overall level of comfort and respiratory status. Although it does not identify degree of confusion, it is useful in defining salient end points and linking treatment to them. Shelly's scale also warrants additional clinical trials.

Most critical care flow sheets include a basic Glasgow Score of level of consciousness: motor activity and confusion based on verbal ability. It might be useful to replace the Glasgow Score on the nursing flow sheet with a scale that more accurately assesses the patient's type and degree of discomfort. By introducing a scale similar to Luer's or Shelly's, the flow sheet would offer a way to compare the patient's discomfort/confusion with the infusion of sedation, vital signs, ventilatory status, and urinary output. Integrating a sedation scale into the flow sheet could simplify documentation and analysis of the sedation strategy.

DAILY WAKE-UP

Sedating agents depress neurologic function, making it impossible to accurately assess the patient's orientation and degree of confusion. Some clinicians decrease the sedating agents daily to perform a neurologic assessment. The sedation is decreased slowly until the patient reaches a Ramsay score of 2 or its equivalent. The nurse then determines the patient's orientation and allows the patient to become better oriented to the environment (Barber, 1995; & Stuart Pharmaceuticals, 1993). This also enables the nurse to determine the patient's inherent respiratory rate and effort.

Daily wake-ups also enable the nurse to determine the minimum dose required to provide sedation. The medication is increased slowly until the defined end point is reached. If the patient reaches this level with a lower dose than was formerly used, there is less risk of unwanted side effects.

Family visits may be timed to coincide with the daily wake-up to promote communication within the family. If the patient shows renewed signs of discomfort, agitation, or confusion, the sedation is increased. A minibolus may be administered to rapidly raise serum blood levels and reach a steady state more rapidly.

DRUG TOLERANCE AND WEANING FROM VENTILATOR

When pulmonary and other organ systems improve to the point that the patient can be weaned from ventilatory support, the level and type of sedation in use must be carefully considered. The ideal weaning practice is to slowly decrease sedation at the same time that ventilatory support is decreased. Because this is a period of increased risk of self-extubation (Pesiri, 1994), sedation must be decreased cautiously, and the patient must be observed closely for signs of renewed agitation.

As the patient becomes more awake, the patient's inherent respiratory rate and effort can be measured, and progress toward extubation is made with reliable indicators of respiratory muscle strength.

Protocols for weaning vary among institutions and among practitioners. Often, the ventilatory mode is changed to an IMV or pressure support so that the patient's inherent expired tidal volume, minute ventilation, and peak flow can be measured. The patient must have a positive gag reflex to protect the airway. The patient should be awake enough to cooperate with instructions related to pulmonary toilet, such as coughing, deep breathing, and use of incentive spirometry. The patient must also be able to generate a negative inspiratory pressure great enough to ensure an acceptable spontaneous tidal volume and minute ventilation. Arterial blood gases confirming adequate oxygenation during the ventilatory weaning are standards of practice.

Five drug-related factors can complicate the gradual withdrawal of mechanical ventilation, including (1) tolerance, (2) prolonged elimination half-life, (3) drug withdrawal, (4) persistence of confusion or agitation, and (5) nutritional deficit.

Tolerance is the brain's response to sedation. After 5 to 7 days of medication, the brain increases production of excitatory neurotransmitters, such as norepinephrine, to counteract the sedating effects of opiates and benzodiazepines (Aitkenhead, 1989; Barber, 1995; Farrell, 1994). This leads to administration of higher than average doses to critically ill patients to achieve an acceptable level of comfort.

To decrease doses of opiates while maintaining acceptable comfort levels, the dose of medication is slowly decreased preparatory to weaning from the ventilatory. In some cases the patient can be treated with an opiate agonist-antagonist such as nalbuphine hydrochloride (Nubain). These agents have fewer sedating and respiratory depressant effects. However, because they possess agonist and antagonist effects on different opiate receptors, they cannot be administered in conjunction with pure opiate agonists, such as morphine, or they may precipitate signs of opiate withdrawal (Barber, 1995).

Prolonged elimination half-lives is the second factor complicating weaning from the ventilator. Because critically ill patients are less able to metabolize and excrete sedating medications, the parent drugs and their active metabolites accumulate in the blood, fatty tissue, and receptor sites. Morphine's half-life can be extended from 4 to 13 hours, that of fentanyl from 5 to 25 hours, and that of propofol from 3 to 30 hours (see Table 9-4).

There is evidence that morphine concentrations in the brain are increased due to hypercapnia and the resulting respiratory acidosis (Aitkenhead, 1989). Because carbon dioxide retention can occur during the weaning process, it is particularly important to watch for signs of increased opiate binding to brain receptor sites, manifested by increasing lethargy and hypoventilation.

As medications are titrated down stores in fat, muscle, and bone are redistributed to the blood and brain, causing resedation. This has been found in patients up to 24 hours after the medication was discontinued (Barber, 1995; Carroll & Magruder, 1993; Harvey, 1996; & Luer, 1995). Opiates, benzodiazepine, and propofol can depress the medullary and pontine regions, which regulate minute ventilation. This can result in a decrease in respiratory rate and volume. Opiates can also depress the respiratory centers in the brainstem, which reduces their sensitivity to carbon dioxide, depressing respiratory drive. These effects are more pronounced in the elderly, and in patients with COPD.

Patients with liver or renal failure must be monitored closely. They metabolize the parent drug and excrete the active metabolite more slowly than the patient with normal liver and kidney function does. The lingering respiratory depressant effects of the drugs can decrease pulmonary parameters, which slow the weaning process.

Sedation scales are particularly important during this period. Usually the physician asks that the patient be brought to a lighter level of sedation. Neurologic assessments document the lightening of sedation, which indicates that respiratory depression is also decreased. If the patient has received long-term sedation with a benzodiazepine, some clinicians prefer to switch the patient to propofol for the final weaning and extubation (Aitkenhead, 1989). The opiates and benzodiazepines are discontinued and a propofol infusion is initiated. The propofol is gradually decreased until the patient is awake, comfortable, and able to follow commands. There should be no signs of hypoventilation.

When all extubation criteria are met, the propofol is discontinued. Ten to fifteen minutes later, the patient is extubated. Vital signs, especially oxygen saturation and respiratory rate, are watched carefully for 24 hours for signs of resedation (Barber, 1995; Stuart Pharmaceuticals, 1993).

The third factor complicating weaning from the ventilator is the possibility of withdrawal symptoms emerging. Patients who receive intravenous sedation for more than 5 to 7 days are at risk of development of signs of withdrawal (Luer, 1995). If opiates are withdrawn too quickly, signs of acute opiate withdrawal may appear. These can include anxiety, restlessness, and sleeplessness; nausea, vomiting, and watery diarrhea; piloerection; and gross large muscle spasms.

Rapid withdrawal of benzodiazepines can cause anxiety, insomnia, elevated blood pressure, tremors, and diaphoresis. Abruptly discontinuing these medications from the elderly patient can lead to hallucinations and agitation.

Rapidly discontinuing propofol after an infusion of more than 5 to 7 days can lead to agitation, confusion, and convulsions. Longer periods of infusion require a more gradual rate of decrease (Stuart Pharmaceuticals, 1993).

To prevent opiate withdrawal, the dose can be decreased by 10% per day. Thus, if a patient received a total of 480 μg of fentanyl over 24 hours (200 μg/hr) the previous day, the current dose would be decreased to 175 μg for 24 hours. This is a conservative approach. Some clinicians recommend decreasing the opiate dose by 20% per day (Luer, 1995).

Rapid withdrawal of benzodiazepines can also elicit acute withdrawal symptoms. These may include anxiety and confusion, seizures, and hallucinations.

The fourth factor complicating ventilatory weaning is the persistence of delirium after the pulmonary disorder has been resolved. The organic syndrome, which causes delirium, is slow to resolve. Abnormal brain function often lasts well after the patient's oxygen transfer has been normalized and will require administration of neuroleptic medications after the patient is weaned. But because haloperidol is not a respiratory or CNS depressant, it will not complicate extubation. Decreasing the dose of a benzodiazepine or an opiate may be necessary to ward against resedation, but continuing haloperidol should not present a problem.

It is important not to discount the effects of poor nutritional status on the patient's ability to be weaned off the respirator. Critically ill patients frequently have low serum albumin levels. Their caloric intake may have been decreased as the result of persistent symptoms such as dyspnea, weakness, fatigue, nausea, or pain. Many critical illnesses impair the ability of the GI tract to absorb nutrients. Intubated patients often have diarrhea, which further impedes intake of calories and vitamins.

Malnourished patients tire more easily when switched to a weaning mode. It is important to begin optimizing the patient's nutritional state from the beginning of the ICU stay. That way, when the pulmonary disorders have improved sufficiently to allow for extubation, the patient will have enough strength to move sufficient air.

After the patient is extubated, dosing regimens are adjusted to a level of comfort and a Ramsay score of 1 to 2 or its equivalent. Medication is administered in accordance with the conscious sedation protocols used for the nonintubated patient. Hemodynamic parameters must still be monitored, and the sedation scale must still be used. The possibility of resedation, even days after extubation, must be borne in mind.

ANTAGONISTS

Antagonists for opiates and benzodiazepines are available as emergency interventions. They are not approved for routine use to accelerate weaning from the sedating medication and must be used with caution because they can precipitate acute withdrawal signs.

Naloxone (Narcan) is a competitive opiate antagonist. It binds readily with opiate receptors in the CNS and spinal cord, driving out opiates. The opiates are then metabolized by the liver and excreted. So long as therapeutic blood levels of Narcan are maintained, opiates will not affect the nervous system.

The therapeutic dose of naloxone is 0.4 to 1.0 mg given intravenously. It has a rapid onset, producing reversal in one minute or less, depending on blood transit times. Because the half-life of opiates in the critically ill patient may be prolonged, the reversing agent may have to be repeated at 0.5- to 1-hour intervals if signs of resedation appear.

Flumazenil (Mazicon) is a benzodiazepine-reversing agent. It has a rapid onset, producing reversal in 1 minute or less. A dose of 0.2 to 1.0 mg is given by a slow intravenous route. The dose should not exceed 0.2 mg/min. Onset is in 1 to 3 minutes, and peak drug levels occur in 6 to 10 minutes.

Flumazenil may be repeated every 20 minutes, with the total dose not exceeding 3 mg/hr. Its serum half-life is 0.6 to 1.3 hours. As with the opiates, the elimination times of benzodiazepines may be prolonged in the ICU. For this reason, it may be necessary to repeat flumazenil. The patient is monitored for resedation. Patients with a history of seizures should be watched closely because flumazenil can lower seizure thresholds.

CONCLUSION

The administration of sedation and analgesia to the critically ill patient involves unique forms of pathophysiologic mechanisms, pharmacokinetics, and modes of drug delivery. The nurse must determine the reason for the patient's anxiety, discomfort, or confusion and initiate appropriate interventions. Nursing responsibilities include monitoring hemodynamic parameters, observing for unwanted side effects, and assessing the effectiveness of the interventions. When administering sedation and analgesia the RN must observe for signs and symptoms of drug accumulation and tolerance. During the weaning phase the RN must safely withdraw the medications while closely observing for signs of drug withdrawal. The recommendations in this chapter will assist the RN managing the care of the critically ill patient receiving sedation and analgesia.

REFERENCES

Aitkenhead, A., Willats, S., Park, G., Collins, C., Ledingham, I., Pepperman, M., Coates, D., Bodenham, A., Smith, M., & Wallace, P. (1989). Comparison of propofol and midazolam for sedation in critically ill patients. *Lancet, .., ..,* 704-709.

Aitkenhead, A. R. (1989). Analgesia and sedation in intensive care. *British Journal of Anesthesia, 63,* 196-206.

American Psychiatric Association (1996). *Diagnostic and statistical manual of mental disorders* (3rd ed.). Washington, DC: Author.

Barber, J. (1995). *Critical care pharmacology* [Seminar]. Barbara Clark Mims Associates.

Bizek, K. (1995). Optimizing sedation in critically ill, mechanically ventilated patients. *Nursing Clinics of North America, 22*(56), 315-324.

Carroll, K., & Magruder, K. (1993). The role of analgesics and sedatives in the management of pain and agitation during weaning from mechanical ventilation. *Critical Care Nurse Quarterly, 15*(4), 68-77.

Crippen, D. (1994). Brain failure in critical care medicine. *Critical Care Nurse Quarterly, 16*(4), 80-95.

Crippen, D., & Ermakov, S. (1992). Stress, agitation and brain failure in critical care medicine. *Critical Care Nurse Quarterly, 15*(2), 52-74.

Farrell, M. (1994). Opiate withdrawal. *Addiction, 89,* 1471-1475.

Geary, S. (1994). Intensive care unit psychosis revisited: Understanding and managing delirium in the critical care setting. *Critical Care Nursing Quarterly, 17*(1), 51-63.

Hansen-Flaschen, J., Cowen, J., & Polomano, R. (1994). Beyond the Ramsay scale: Need for a validated measure of sedating drug efficacy in the intensive care unit. *Critical Care Medicine, 22*(5), 732-733.

Harper, J. (1994). Need for a validated measure of sedating drug efficacy. *Critical Care Medicine, 23*(2), 417-418.

Harvey, M. (1996). Managing agitation in critically ill patients. *American Journal of Critical Care, 5*(1), 7-15.

Jensen, D., & Justic, M. (1995). An algorithm to distinguish the need for sedative, anxiolytic and analgesic agents. *Dimensions of Critical Care Nursing, 14*(2), 58-69.

Kosten, T., & McCance, E. (1996). A review of pharmacotherapies for substance abuse. *American Journal of Addictions, 5*(1), 58-63.

Luer, J. (1995). Sedation and chemical relaxation in critical pulmonary illness: Suggestions for patient assessment and drug monitoring. *AACN Clinical Issues, 6*(2), 333-343.

Murray, M. (1994). Analgesia in the critically ill patient. *New Horizons, 2*(1), 56-63.

Pasero, C. (1994). Avoiding opioid-induced respiratory depression. *American Journal of Nursing, 94* (4), 25-31.

Pesiri, A. (1994). Two-year study of the prevention of unintentional extubation. *Critical Care Nurse Quarterly, 17*(3), 35-39.

Riker, R., Gilles, F., & Cox, P. (1994). Continuous infusion of haloperidol controls agitation in critically ill patients, *Critical Care Medicine, 22*(3), 433-440.

Shapiro, B., Greenbaum, D., Schein, R., Warren, J., Egol, A., Jacobi, J., Nasraway, S., Spevetz, A., & Stonde, J. (1995). Practice parameters for intravenous analgesia and sedation for adult patients in the intensive care unit: An executive summary. *Critical Care Medicine, 21*(9), 1596-1599.

Shelly, M. (1994). Assessing sedation. *Care of the Critically Ill, 10*(3), 118-121.

Stern, T. (1994). Continuous infusion of haloperidol in agitated, critically ill patients. *Critical Care Medicine, 22*(3), 378-379.

Stuart Pharmaceuticals (1993). Propofol: A physician's guide to use in the intensive care unit. Wilmington, DE: Author.

Vitello, J. M., Harvey, M., Pine, L., Searle, L., Thomas, K., Ramsay, M., Davidson, J. (1996). Management of sedation: the nursing perspective. *Critical Care Nurse/Supplement,* 16 (4 Suppl), 1-14; quiz 15-6.

Wheeler, A. (1993). Sedation, analgesia, and paralysis in the intensive care unit. *Chest, 104*(2), 566-569.

State Boards of Nursing Positions on Conscious Sedation

ARKANSAS STATE BOARD OF NURSING

POSITION STATEMENT 94-1: ADMINISTRATION OF INTRAVENOUS CONSCIOUS SEDATION BY THE REGISTERED NURSE*

The Arkansas State Board of Nursing has determined that it is within the scope of practice of a registered professional nurse to administer pharmacologic agents by the intravenous route to produce conscious sedation. Optimal anesthesia care is best provided by qualified anesthesiologists and certified registered nurse anesthetists. However, the Board recognizes that the demand in the practice setting necessitates noncertified registered nurse- anesthetist RNs providing intravenous conscious sedation.

Employing facilities should have policies and procedures to guide the RN. The attached guidelines have been adopted by the Arkansas State Board of Nursing (see Appendix C).

CALIFORNIA BOARD OF REGISTERED NURSING

INTRAVENOUS SEDATION†

It is within the scope of practice of registered nurses to administer intravenous medications for the purpose of induction of conscious sedation for short-term therapeutic, diagnostic, or surgical procedures.

Authority for RNs to administer medication derives from § 2725(b) of the Nursing Practice Act (NPA). This section places no limits on the type of medication or route of administration; there is only a requirement that the drug be ordered by one lawfully authorized to prescribe. Other relevant sections of the NPA do impose additional requirements. Specifically, the RN must be competent to perform the function, and the function must be performed in a manner consistent with the standard of practice (Business and Professions Code 2761(a)(1), California Code of Regulations 1442, 1443, 1443.5.).

---

*Board action November 1994. Reprinted with permission.
†September 1995. Reprinted with permission.

In administering medications to induce conscious sedation, the RN is required to have the same knowledge and skills as for any other medication the nurse administers. This knowledge base includes but is not limited to effects of medications, potential side effects of the medication, contraindications for the administration of the medication, and the amount of the medication to be administered. The requisite skills include the ability to competently and safely administer the medication by the specified route, anticipate and recognize potential complications of the medication, recognize emergency situations, and institute emergency procedures. Thus the RN would be held accountable for knowledge of the medication and for ensuring that the proper safety measures are followed. National guidelines for administering conscious sedation should be consulted in establishing agency policies and procedures.

The RN administering agents to render conscious sedation would conduct a nursing assessment to determine that administration of the drug is in the patient's best interest. The RN would also ensure that all safety measures are in force, including backup personnel skilled and trained in airway management, resuscitation, and emergency intubation, should complications occur. RNs managing the care of patients receiving intravenous conscious sedation shall not leave the patient unattended or engage in tasks that would compromise continuous monitoring of the patient by the RN. RN functions as described in this policy may not be assigned to unlicensed assistive personnel.

The RN is held accountable for any act of nursing provided to a client. The RN has the right and obligation to act as the client's advocate by refusing to administer or continue to administer any medication not in the client's best interest; this includes medications which would render the client's level of sedation to deep sedation and/or loss of consciousness. The institution should have in place a process for evaluating and documenting the RNs demonstration of knowledge, skills, and abilities for the management of clients receiving agents to render conscious sedation. Evaluation and documentation of competency should occur on a periodic basis.

Certified registered nurse anesthetists by virtue of advanced education and practice in their area of specialty have met requirements to administer safely the class of drugs in question.

Addendum: Intravenous Sedation

As of 1995, safety considerations for intravenous sedation include continuous monitoring of oxygen saturation, cardiac rate and rhythm, blood pressure, respiratory rate, and level of consciousness, as specified in national guidelines or standards. Immediate availability of emergency care which contains resuscitative and antagonist medications, airway and ventilatory adjunct equipment, defibrillator, suction, and a source for administration of 100% oxygen are commonly included in national standards for inducing conscious sedation.

RESOURCES

AORN recommended practices for monitoring the patient receiving intravenous sedation. Association of Operating Room Nurses, Inc., 2170 S Parker Road, Denver, CO 80231; telephone (303) 755-6300.

Position statement on the role of the registered nurse in the management of patients receiving IV conscious sedation for short-term therapeutic, diagnostic, or surgical procedures (endorsed by 23 professional associations). American Nurses Association, 600 Maryland Ave. S.W., Suite 100 W., Washington, DC 20024-2571; telephone (202) 554-4444.

Qualified providers of conscious sedation. American Association of Nurse Anesthetists, 222 S. Prospect Ave., Park Ridge, IL 60068; telephone (708) 692-7050.

IDAHO STATE BOARD OF NURSING

MEDICATION ADMINISTRATION TO PRODUCE AN ANESTHESIA EFFECT: OCTOBER 1985*

RNs may not legally administer medications, singly or in combination, when such medications are given for the purpose of producing anesthesia, as anesthesia care services must be provided by certified RN anesthetists.

DEFINITIONS ANESTHESIA/HYPNOSIS: FEBRUARY 1986*

The following decisions were approved:

Anesthesia—The administration of reversible drugs given for the purpose of rendering the individual unconscious and unsusceptible to pain.

Hypnosis—The induction of a trancelike state of dissociation and altered consciousness that includes sensory, motor, and psychological changes; an altered state of awareness, perception, and memory; and/or a state of acute awareness and directed attention, which results in increased responsiveness to suggestion.

IOWA BOARD OF NURSING

DECLARATORY RULING NO. 36: REGISTERED NURSES ADMINISTERING INTRAVENOUS VERSED [MIDAZOLAM HYDROCHLORIDE]*

Petitions for reconsideration of Declaratory Ruling No. 32 were filed with the Iowa Board of Nursing by Linda Fennelly, RN, Director, Medical/Surgical Nursing, St. Luke's Hospital, Davenport, Iowa, and Peg A. Mehmert, RN, Assistant Director: Nursing Systems and Research, Mercy Hospital, Davenport, Iowa, on January 4, 1989, and December 14, 1988.

---

*Reprinted with permission.

Based on information received by the Board, Declaratory Ruling No. 32 is rescinded and this ruling is substituted in its place.

Questions presented in the original petition were:

1. In the acute and skilled care units of St. Luke's Hospital, Davenport, Iowa, may RNs administer Versed via continuous intravenous drip and/or by intravenous push under the written order of a physician?

2. May RNs employed by St. Luke's Home Care administer intravenous Versed via continuous drip and/or by intravenous push to a terminally ill patient once the patient is stabilized in the hospital setting and the medication is used as adjuvant therapy along with a narcotic for pain control?

3. If RNs are not permitted to administer intravenous Versed, may they:
   a. Teach the patient or significant other to self-administer?
   b. When a change in prescription occurs, go to the patient's home and adjust the pump setting of the infusion control device?

The questions presented in the request for reconsideration are:

1. May an RN employed at Mercy Hospital or St. Luke's Hospital in Davenport, Iowa, administer the first dose of intravenous Versed and titrate the dose on the order of a physician?

2. May an RN administer intravenous Versed via a continuous drip to any patient, regardless of whether a patient is terminally ill, on the order of a physician?

3. Does a patient require continuous monitoring while receiving intravenous Versed?

The Board is authorized to issue declaratory rulings "as to the applicability of any statutory provision, rule or other written statement of law or policy, decision, or order of the agency" pursuant to Iowa Code §17A.9 (1987). *See also* Iowa Administrative Code, Nursing Board (655), Chapter 9.

The facts leading to the original request were as follows:

> A terminally ill patient at St. Luke's Hospital in Davenport, Iowa, was receiving high-dose narcotics to control his pain. His use of narcotics diminished significantly when the narcotics were administered intrathecally along with intravenous Versed on a continuous drip.

The facts leading to the request for reconsideration include:

- It was the intent of St. Luke's Hospital that RNs be permitted to administer intravenous Versed via continuous drip to any patient on an acute or skilled nursing unit as ordered by the physician, and not limit administration to only terminally ill patients.

- A Versed drip may be ordered at any time as adjunct to pain control and a physician will not always be available to administer an initial dose or be able to remain with a patient for several hours while the dose is titrated.

- Continuous monitoring of a patient receiving intravenous Versed presents an ethical dilemma for those terminally ill patients who have "do not resuscitate" orders.
- RNs in the endoscopy suite at Mercy Hospital had been administering the initial and subsequent doses of intravenous push Versed on the order of a physician.

Nursing responsibilities in delivering home and hospital care would include:

1. Patient assessment
2. Patient education, drug administration, care of access device, operating the pump, self-monitoring, and observing for side effects
3. Administering the medication and teaching pharmacologic action, dosage range, side effects, and clinical monitoring
4. Continuing patient monitoring by regularly scheduled and "on-call" home visits
5. Catheter site care
6. Operation of the infusion device (set up and reprogramming)
7. Emergency procedures related to central venous access device dislodgment or drug-related adverse reactions

Versed is a short-acting benzodiazepine central nervous system depressant. The following warning is printed in the Roche Laboratories guidelines:

> Versed must never be used without individualization of dosage. Prior to the intravenous administration of Versed in any dose, the immediate availability of oxygen, resuscitative equipment and skilled personnel for the maintenance of a patent airway and support of ventilation should be ensured. Patient should be continuously monitored for early signs of underventilation or apnea, which can lead to hypoxia/cardiac arrest unless effective counter measures are taken immediately.

The Board of Nursing considered the administration of intravenous Versed to a patient via continuous drip and/or intravenous push to be within the scope of practice of an RN in an acute and skilled care unit of St. Luke's Hospital and Mercy Hospital, Davenport, Iowa, and not within the scope of practice of an RN in a home care setting. The RN may teach the patient and family members self-administration and pump setting adjustment in a home setting. The RN employed in a home setting may not adjust the pump setting of the infusion control device.

Rationale

Iowa Administrative Code, Nursing Board [655],§ 6.2(5) states in part:

> The registered nurse shall recognize and understand the legal implications of accountability. Accountability includes but not need be limited to the following:
> a. Performing or supervising those activities and functions which require the knowledge and skill level currently ascribed to the registered nurse and seeking assistance when activities and functions are beyond the licensee's scope of preparation.

The RN in an acute and skilled care unit of St. Luke's Hospital or Mercy Hospital, Davenport, Iowa, has immediate availability of oxygen, resuscitative equipment, and skilled personnel for maintenance of a patent airway and support of ventilation. This is not available in a home setting and therefore the nurse cannot assure safe delivery of nursing care. If the patient is willing to assume the risk of self-administration of the medication then the RN may teach those skills to the patient and the family members.

In an acute and skilled care unit of St. Luke's Hospital and Mercy Hospital, the RN may administer intravenous Versed via continuous drip and/or intravenous push if the following conditions are met:

1. Initial administration and titration of medication may be performed by an RN on the order of a physician.
2. There must be immediate availability of oxygen, resuscitative equipment, and skilled personnel for the maintenance of a patent airway.
3. The patient will be monitored for signs of underventilation or apnea.
4. The institution has a written policy identifying that the procedure is acceptable practice for the RN in the facility.
5. The procedure has been prescribed by the physician by a written order.

REFERENCE

Versed dosage and administration guidelines. (1988). Roche Laboratories.

CONSULTANTS

C. J. Cronshey, Product Service Manager, Roche Laboratories, Nutley, New Jersey.
Barbara Rodts, RN, BSN, Visiting Nurse Association, Davenport, Iowa.

LOUISIANA STATE BOARD OF NURSING

LOUISIANA STATE BOARD OF NURSING STATEMENT ON CONSCIOUS SEDATION*

In reference to Agenda Item #7, conscious sedation is defined as a state of mild to moderate sedation permitting cooperation and tolerance of diagnostic and therapeutic medical procedures.

The administration of intravenous conscious sedation is within the realm of practice of an RN provided the following conditions are met:

1. The physician must be present.
2. The patient must be adequately monitored according to currently recognized standards of practice.

---

*Adopted September 20, 1990. Reprinted with permission.

3. The RN must constantly observe and monitor the patient.
4. The institution must have a policy which addresses:
   a. Maximum dosage which may be administered by the RN for the purpose of intravenous conscious sedation during medical procedures.
   b. Resources which must be immediately available, including, but not limited to, resuscitative equipment and resuscitative personnel.
5. There is a specific written medical order, signed by the physician, for each patient receiving the treatment.
6. The patient has a patent intravenous access.
7. The manufacturer's guidelines are followed.
8. There is documentation that the RN has the necessary knowledge and skills to perform the procedure.
9. The administration of medications for conscious sedation is according to currently accepted nursing standards of practice.

MARYLAND BOARD OF NURSING

DECLARATORY RULING 93-3, SEPTEMBER 28, 1993: REGISTERED NURSE ADMINISTRATION OF CONSCIOUS SEDATION FOR SHORT-TERM THERAPEUTIC, DIAGNOSTIC, AND SURGICAL PROCEDURES*

By letter dated November 22, 1992, Phyllis Sanford, LPN, President, Chesapeake Society of Gastroenterology Nurses and Association, asked the Maryland Board of Nursing whether an RN may administer intravenous conscious sedation for a client receiving diagnostic or surgical procedure.

The Board is authorized to issue declaratory rulings pursuant to State Government Article 10-301 et seq. and the Maryland Board of Nursing Regulations found at COMAR 10.27.08 governing Issuance of Petitions for a Declaratory Ruling.

Board Ruling

For the purpose of clarity, the term *conscious sedation* has been defined in order that it can be differentiated from other sedative medications that all licensed nurses routinely administer.

Conscious sedation is a minimally depressed level of consciousness that allows the client to retain the ability to maintain a patent airway independently and continuously and to respond appropriately to physical stimulation and/or verbal command. Conscious sedation may be easily converted into a state of deep sedation or loss of consciousness because of the unique characteristics of the drugs used, as well

---

*Reprinted with permission.

as other factors indicating the physical status and drug sensitivities of the individual client. The administration of conscious sedation requires continuous monitoring of the client and the ability to respond immediately to any deviation from normal.

Given the above-noted definition, the Board has determined that it is within the scope of practice of an RN to administer and monitor intravenous conscious sedation for a client undergoing a diagnostic and/or surgical procedure only when the following specific conditions are met:

1. Medications must be ordered by only a physician or dentist, who must be immediately available in the room during the diagnostic and/or surgical procedure.

2. The employer must have in place an educational/credentialing mechanism which includes a process for evaluating and documenting the RN's demonstration of the knowledge, skills, and abilities related to the management of clients receiving intravenous conscious sedation. Evaluation and documentation of competency should occur on a periodic basis.

3. To be qualified, the RN managing the care of the client receiving intravenous conscious sedation must:

   a. Demonstrate the acquired knowledge of anatomy, physiology, pharmacology, cardiac arrhythmia recognition, and complications related to intravenous conscious sedation and medications.

   b. Possess the requisite knowledge and skills to assess and intervene, in the event of complications or undesired outcomes, and to institute appropriate nursing interventions.

   c. Possess current Basic Life Support certification.

4. The registered nurse administering the IV conscious sedation must have the primary responsibilities for monitoring the client during the procedure and may not leave the client unattended or engage in tasks that would compromise continuous monitoring.

5. All clients receiving intravenous conscious sedation must have a patent intravenous access maintained from the beginning of medication administration until recovery from conscious sedation.

6. Supplemental oxygen must be available to all clients receiving intravenous conscious sedation per order (including standing orders).

7. All clients receiving intravenous conscious sedation must be continuously monitored throughout the procedure by oxygen saturation, cardiac rate and rhythm, blood pressure, respiratory rate, level of consciousness and according to currently recognized national nursing professional standards.

8. All clients receiving intravenous conscious sedation must be continuously monitored throughout the recovery phase, by blood pressure, pulse, and respiratory status and according to currently recognized national nursing professional specialty standards.

9. An emergency cart must be immediately accessible to every location where intravenous conscious sedation is administered. This cart must include at least the following: emergency resuscitative and antagonist drugs, airway and ventilatory adjunct equipment, defibrillator, and a source for administration of 100% oxygen. An Ambu/PMR bag, oxygen, and appropriate airways must be in each room where intravenous conscious sedation is administered.

10. The employer must maintain a written protocol for the procedure which includes, but is not limited to:
    a. All the previous requirements
    b. Provisions for back-up personnel who are Advanced Cardiac Life Support certified and who are expert in airway management and emergency intubation, should complications arise

Concluding Statement

The RN is responsible and accountable for all actions/lack of action that he/she takes when administering and/or monitoring the client receiving conscious sedation. The RN is required to have the same knowledge base for the medications administered to induce conscious sedation and for any other medication that he/she administers. This knowledge base includes, but is not limited to:

1. Effect of the medication
2. Potential side effects of the medication
3. Contraindications of the administration of the medication
4. The amount of the medication to be administered at any one time (includes initial dose, maintenance dose, and total amount of the medication administered for the procedure).
5. Ability to anticipate and recognize potential complications of the medication
6. Ability to recognize emergency situations and institute appropriate nursing interventions

While the RN who administers intravenous conscious sedation is acting on a specific physician's order for a specific client, the RN has the right and the obligation to refuse to administer and/or continue to administer medication(s) in amounts which may convert the client's state to deep sedation and/or loss of consciousness.

As this specialized procedure requires specialized education, training, and nursing judgment, the RN is held accountable to refuse to perform this specialized act or any other act of nursing which is beyond the parameters of the licensee's education, capabilities, and experience.

It is inappropriate, unacceptable, and in violation of Health Occupations Article, Title 8, for an RN who is not a Maryland Board of Nursing–Certified RN Anesthetist to administer drugs classified as anesthetics, including, but not limited to, ketamine, sodium thiopental, methohexital, propofol, etomidate, and nitrous oxide.

MONTANA BOARD OF NURSING

*DECLARATORY RULING**

In the matter of the petition for declaratory ruling on the administration of intravenous conscious sedation medications by non-anesthetist registered nurses.

Introduction

1. On October 13, 1994, the Board of Nursing published a Notice of Petition for Declaratory Ruling in the above-entitled matter at page 2752, 1994 Montana Administrative Register, issue number 19.
2. On November 7, 1994, the Board presided over a hearing in this matter to consider written and oral testimony from interested individuals.
3. After consideration of the testimony and deliberation, the Board passed a motion to grant the petition for declaratory ruling.

Issue

4. Petitioners requested a ruling on whether it is within the scope of practice of a non-anesthetist RN to administer intravenous conscious sedation medications under a physician's order based on the Board's interpretation of § 37-8-102(5) (b), MCA, defining professional nursing.

Factual Background

5. The Petitioners represent the nursing staff at the Kalispell Regional Hospital and set forth the following definition of "intravenous conscious sedation" as adopted by the Association of Operating Room Nurses (AORN):

    Intravenous conscious sedation is produced by the administration of pharmacologic agents. A patient under conscious sedation has a depressed level of consciousness but retains the ability to independently and continuously maintain a patent airway and respond appropriately to physical stimulation and/or verbal command.

6. The Petition alleges that non-anesthetist RNs currently perform intravenous conscious sedation for short-term therapeutic, surgical, or diagnostic procedures, and that this practice provides cost-effective, quality healthcare.
7. The Petitioners requested this declaratory ruling to clarify that intravenous conscious sedation is within the scope of a non-anesthetist RN who has had specialized training pursuant to a written standard of care describing con-

---

*Reprinted with permission.

scious sedation policies and procedures as required by the Joint Commission on Hospital Accreditation.

Summary of Comments

8. Kate Triplett, RN, submitted written testimony against allowing non-anesthetist RNs to administer intravenous conscious sedation, expressing the need for RNs performing the procedure to have specialized knowledge for anesthetic agents and potential side effects. Ms. Triplett further expressed the need for immediate accessibility to monitoring equipment, intubation equipment, and oxygen supplies when intravenous conscious sedation is being performed.

9. Several nurses signed their names to written statements submitted on behalf of Saint Vincent's Hospital and Health Center and Deaconess Medical Center in support of the petition. The testimony indicated that it is common practice for non-anesthetist nurses to administer intravenous conscious sedation under a physician's order. Both facilities follow the AORN standards of care with regard to administration of intravenous conscious sedation. These standards include parameters to be assessed during procedures which indicate a need for intravenous conscious sedation and a patient-monitoring policy.

10. The Montana Nurses' Association, represented by Barbard Booher, testified in support of the petition. This testimony included a position statement adopting the AORN standard of care with regard to the role of the RN in administering intravenous conscious sedation.

Relevant Law

11. The scope of practice of an RN is set forth at § 37-8-102(5) (b), MCA, and includes "the administration of medications and treatments prescribed by physicians. . . ."

12. ARM 8.32.1404(2) and (3) state that the RN shall "accept responsibility for individual nursing actions and competence and base practice on validated data" and shall "obtain instruction and supervision as necessary when implementing nursing techniques or practices."

Conclusion

13. Based on these definitions, rules, statutes, and the facts herein cited, the Board of Nursing adopts the position that it is within the scope of practice of a non-anesthetist RN to administer intravenous conscious sedation medication.

The Petition is granted. DATED this 11th day of January, 1995.

NORTH CAROLINA BOARD OF NURSING

THE ROLE OF THE REGISTERED NURSE IN THE MANAGEMENT OF PATIENTS RECEIVING INTRAVENOUS CONSCIOUS SEDATION*

Definition of Intravenous Conscious Sedation

> Intravenous conscious sedation is produced by the administration of pharmacologic agents. The patient under conscious sedation has a depressed level of consciousness but retains the ability to independently and continuously maintain a patent airway and respond appropriately to physical stimulation and/or verbal command (American Nurses Association, *SCI Nursing,* June 1992).

Use of intravenous conscious sedation is becoming more common in a variety of practice settings. The RN who is asked to administer pharmaceutical agents and monitor the patient during the course of the sedated period must consider the following aspects of nursing care *prior to* accepting these responsibilities for a patient requiring intravenous conscious sedation. The NCAC 21:36.0224—Components of Nursing Practice for the Registered Nurse (a) (1-6) states:

> The responsibilities which any registered nurse can safely accept are determined by the variables in each nursing practice setting. These variables include:
>
> (1) the nurse's own qualifications including:
>   (a) basic educational preparation; and
>   (b) knowledge and skills subsequently acquired through continuing education and practice;
> (2) the complexity and frequency of nursing care needed by a given client population;
> (3) the proximity of clients to personnel;
> (4) the qualifications and number of staff;
> (5) the accessible resources; and
> (6) established policies, procedures, practices, and channels of communication which lend support to the types of nursing services offered.

NCAC 21:36.0221 (c) (1)—License Required—describes the accountability of the RN for medication administration as follows:

> The nurse who assumes responsibility for implementing a treatment and pharmaceutical regimen is accountable for:
>
> (a) recognizing side effects;
> (b) recognizing toxic effects;
> (c) recognizing allergic reactions;
> (d) recognizing immediate desired effects;
> (e) recognizing unusual and unexpected effects;
> (f) recognizing changes in client's condition that contraindicate continued administration of the medications;

---

*Reprinted with permission.

(g) anticipating those effects which may rapidly endanger a client's life or well-being; and

(h) making judgments and decisions concerning actions to take in the event such untoward effects occur.

In-depth knowledge of anatomy, physiology, pharmacology, patient assessment, and emergency procedures are necessary for the RN to accept responsibility for monitoring the client receiving intravenous conscious sedation.

Accessible resources include equipment, such as pulse oximeter and cardiac monitors, as well as personnel. In an outpatient setting, for example, an RN who has the appropriate knowledge and skills, may accept the responsibility for managing the patient receiving intravenous conscious sedation provided the agency has written policies and procedures which support this activity. Personnel qualified to provide necessary emergency measures, such as intubation and airway management, must be readily available. Emergency procedures such as endotracheal intubation and defibrillation are Category II activities for the RN only.

Therefore, the RN may accept the responsibility for the care of patients receiving intravenous conscious sedation if he/she has the appropriate knowledge and skills and is in a practice setting that provides the necessary resources to assure patient safety. This management may include administration of medications, monitoring the patient for intended and untoward responses to the medication and his/her level of consciousness throughout the procedure, and implementing emergency activities (e.g., endotracheal intubation and defibrillation), if required. The RN who accepts the responsibility of monitoring the status of the patient cannot assume other responsibilities which would leave the client unattended, thereby jeopardizing the safety of the client. Given the level of knowledge and skill required, as well as the need for independent decision-making, nursing management of these patients is *beyond* the LPN scope of practice.

Specific guidelines for the RN's preparation and role in managing patients receiving intravenous conscious sedation have been developed by both the ANA and a consortium of national professional nursing organizations and may be obtained directly from the ANA at 600 Maryland Ave., S.W., Suite 100 W., Washington, DC 20024-2571. You may also contact a practice consultant at the Board Office to discuss nursing law as it relates to this area of practice.

NORTH DAKOTA BOARD OF NURSING

OPINION[*]

In the opinion of the North Dakota Board of Nursing, it is appropriate for an RN with the necessary knowledge, skills, and abilities to be responsible for monitoring

---

[*]June 8, 1990. Reprinted with permission.

patients receiving sedative medications for diagnostic or special procedures if the following conditions are met:

1. The RN's primary responsibility is monitoring the patient's condition.
2. Appropriate equipment for monitoring and resuscitation is immediately available and the RN is prepared to use that equipment (which includes, at a minimum, pulse oximetry, noninvasive blood pressure, electrocardiogram).
3. The agency has written policies in place addressing:
   a. supervisory requirements and credentials review for those RNs assigned to monitor patients receiving sedative medication.
   b. the requirement for constant attendance until the patient is fully responsive or has recovered protective reflexes.
   c. procedures for administration, monitoring, documentation, and emergency resuscitation for patients receiving sedative medication.

SOUTH CAROLINA BOARD OF NURSING

QUESTION*

Is it within the role and scope of responsibilities of the RN to administer pharmacologic agents intravenously for preoperative and conscious sedation?

Advisory Opinion

The Board of Nursing for South Carolina acknowledges that it is within the role and scope of the responsibilities of the RN to administer medications for preoperative sedation and conscious sedation as ordered by a licensed physician or dentist.

The Board recommends that if the nursing services component of the respective employing agency determines that implementation is in order, then appropriate policies, procedures, and protocols should be developed which specify patient situations in which the RN is authorized to administer intravenous drugs for preoperative and conscious sedation, to include dose ranges and precautions for specific drugs.

The opinion statement is an advisory opinion of the Board of Nursing as to what constitutes competence and safe nursing practice.

REFERENCE

Position statement on the role of the registered nurse (RN) in the management of patients receiving IV conscious sedation for short-term therapeutic, diagnostic, or surgical procedures, November 1, 1991. (See Appendix C.)

---

*Formulated May 18, 1989. Reviewed January 1990–March 1992. Revised July 1993.

SOUTH DAKOTA BOARD OF NURSING

DECLARATORY RULING 89-1*

Although RNs, under the direction of a physician, may administer narcotics, analgesics, sedatives, and tranquilizing medications to patients, RNs may not administer any medication for the purpose of inducing general anesthesia. It is not within the authority of the board to determine how or for what purpose a specific drug with multiple uses is being administered at any given time. Institutional or agency protocol must address this.

BOARD OF NURSE EXAMINERS FOR THE STATE OF TEXAS

POSITION STATEMENT 15.8: ADMINISTRATION OF INTRAVENOUS CONSCIOUS SEDATION BY THE REGISTERED NURSE†

The Board has determined that it is within the scope of practice of a registered professional nurse to administer pharmacologic agents via the intravenous route to produce conscious sedation. Optimal anesthesia care is best provided by qualified anesthesiologists and certified registered nurse-anesthetists; however, the Board recognizes that the demand in the practice setting necessitates non–certified registered nurse-anesthetist RNs providing intravenous conscious sedation.

Employing facilities should have policies and procedures to guide the RN. The professional associations, including the American Nurses Association and the American Association of Nurse Anesthetists, provide excellent guidelines.

STATE OF WISCONSIN DEPARTMENT OF REGULATION AND LICENSING

BOARD OF NURSING, CHAPTER N 6, WISCONSIN ADMINISTRATIVE CODE‡

§ N 6.03(2), Code

  (2) Performance of Delegated Medical Acts. In the performance of delegated medical acts an RN shall:

    (a) Accept only those delegated medical acts for which there are protocols or written or verbal orders;

    (b) Accept only those delegated medical acts for which the RN is competent to perform based on his or her nursing education, training, or experience;

    (c) Consult with a physician, dentist, or podiatrist in cases where the RN knows or should know a delegated medical act may harm a patient; and

    (d) Perform delegated medical acts under the general supervision or direction of a physician, dentist, or podiatrist.

---

*Reprinted with permission.
†Board action, January 1992.
‡Reprinted with permission.

American Society of Anesthesiologists Standards for Basic Anesthetic Monitoring*

These standards apply to all anesthesia care although in emergency circumstances appropriate life support measures take precedence. These standards may be exceeded at any time based on the judgment of the responsible anesthesiologist. They are intended to encourage quality patient care, but observing them cannot guarantee any specific patient outcome. They are subject to revision from time to time, as warranted by the evolution of technology and practice. They apply to all general anesthetics, regional anesthetics, and monitored anesthesia care. This set of standards addresses only the issue of basic anesthetic monitoring, which is one component of anesthesia care. In certain rare or unusual circumstances (1) some of these methods of monitoring may be clinically impractical and (2) appropriate use of the described monitoring methods may fail to detect untoward clinical developments. Brief interruptions of continual[†] monitoring may be unavoidable. Under extenuating circumstances, the responsible anesthesiologist may waive the requirements marked with an asterisk (*); it is recommended that when this is done, it should be so stated (including the reasons) in a note in the patient's medical record. These standards are not intended for application to the care of the obstetric patient in labor or in the conduct of pain management.

STANDARD I

Qualified anesthesia personnel shall be present in the room throughout the conduct of all general anesthetics, regional anesthetics, and monitored anesthesia care.

Standards for Basic Anesthetic Monitoring (ASA Directory of Members 1995, pp. 384-385) is reprinted with permission of the American Society of Anesthesiologists, 520 N. Northwest Highway, Park Ridge, IL 60068-2573.
*Approved by American Society of Anesthesiologists House of Delegates on October 21, 1986; last amended on October 13, 1993.
†Note that *continual* is defined as "repeated regularly and frequently in steady rapid succession," whereas *continuous* means "prolonged without any interruption at any time."

OBJECTIVE

Because of the rapid changes in patient status during anesthesia, qualified anesthesia personnel shall be continuously present to monitor the patient and provide anesthesia care. In the event there is a direct known hazard (e.g., radiation) to the anesthesia personnel which might require intermittent remote observation of the patient, some provision for monitoring the patient must be made. In the event that an emergency requires the temporary absence of the person primarily responsible for the anesthetic, the best judgment of the anesthesiologist will be exercised in comparing the emergency with the anesthetized patient's condition and in the selection of the person left responsible for the anesthetic during the temporary absence.

STANDARD II

During administration of all anesthetics, the patient's oxygenation, ventilation, circulation, and temperature shall be continually evaluated.

OXYGENATION
Objective

To ensure adequate oxygen concentration in the inspired gas and the blood during all anesthetics.

Methods

1. *Inspired gas:* During every administration of general anesthesia with an anesthesia machine, the concentration of oxygen in the patient breathing system shall be measured by an oxygen analyzer with a low oxygen concentration limit alarm in use.*
2. *Blood oxygenation:* During administration of all anesthetics, a quantitative method of assessing oxygenation such as pulse oximetry shall be employed.* Adequate illumination and exposure of the patient are necessary to assess color.*

VENTILATION
Objective

To ensure adequate ventilation of the patient during all anesthetics.

Methods

1. Every patient receiving general anesthesia shall have the adequacy of ventilation continually evaluated. While qualitative clinical signs such as chest excursion, observation of the reservoir breathing bag, and auscultation of breath sounds may be adequate, quantitative monitoring of the carbon dioxide content and/or volume of expired gas is encouraged.

2. When an endotracheal tube is inserted, its correct positioning in the trachea must be verified by clinical assessment and by identification of carbon dioxide in the expired gas.* End-tidal carbon dioxide analysis, in use from the time of endotracheal tube placement, is strongly encouraged.
3. When ventilation is controlled by a mechanical ventilator, there shall be in continuous use a device that is capable of detecting disconnection of components of the breathing system. The device must give an audible signal when its alarm threshold is exceeded.
4. During regional anesthesia and monitored anesthesia care, the adequacy of ventilation shall be evaluated, at least by continual observation of qualitative clinical signs.

CIRCULATION
Objective
To ensure the adequacy of the patient's circulatory function during administration of all anesthetics.

Methods
1. Every patient receiving anesthesia shall have the electrocardiogram continuously displayed from the beginning of anesthesia until preparing to leave the anesthetizing location.*
2. Every patient receiving anesthesia shall have arterial blood pressure and heart rate determined and evaluated at least every 5 minutes.*
3. Every patient receiving general anesthesia shall have, in addition to the above, circulatory function continually evaluated by at least one of the following: palpitation of a pulse, auscultation of heart sounds, monitoring of a tracing of intra-arterial pressure, ultrasound peripheral pulse monitoring, or pulse plethysmography or oximetry.

BODY TEMPERATURE
Objective
To aid in the maintenance of appropriate body temperature during administration of all anesthetics.

Methods
There shall be readily available a means to continuously measure the patient's temperature. When changes in body temperature are intended, anticipated, or suspected, the temperature shall be measured.

Position Statement on the Role of the Registered Nurse (RN) in the Management of Patients Receiving Intravenous Conscious Sedation for Short-Term Therapeutic, Diagnostic, or Surgical Procedures

DEFINITION OF INTRAVENOUS CONSCIOUS SEDATION

Intravenous conscious sedation is produced by the administration of pharmacologic agents. A patient under conscious sedation has a depressed level of consciousness but retains the ability to independently and continuously maintain a patent airway and respond appropriately to physical stimulation and/or verbal command.

MANAGEMENT AND MONITORING

It is within the scope of practice of a registered nurse to manage the care of patients receiving intravenous conscious sedation during therapeutic, diagnostic, or surgical procedures provided the following criteria are met:

1. Administration of intravenous conscious sedation medications by non-anesthetist RNs is allowed by state laws and institutional policy, procedures, and protocol.
2. A qualified anesthesia provider or attending physician selects and orders the medications to achieve intravenous conscious sedation.
3. Guidelines for patient monitoring, drug administration, and protocols for dealing with potential complications or emergency situations are available and have been developed in accordance with accepted standards of anesthesia practice.
4. The RN managing the care of the patient receiving intravenous conscious sedation shall have no other responsibilities that would leave the patient unattended or compromise continuous monitoring.
5. The RN managing the care of patients receiving intravenous conscious sedation is able to:
   a. Demonstrate the acquired knowledge of anatomy, physiology, pharmacology, cardiac arrhythmia recognition, and complications related to intravenous conscious sedation and medications.
   b. Assess total patient care requirements during intravenous conscious sedation and recovery. Physiologic measurements should include, but not be limited to, respiratory rate, oxygen saturation, blood pressure, cardiac rate and rhythm, and patient's level of consciousness.

    c. Understand the principles of oxygen delivery, respiratory physiology, transport and uptake, and demonstrate the ability to use oxygen delivery devices.

    d. Anticipate and recognize potential complications of intravenous conscious sedation in relation to the type of medication being administered.

    e. Possess the requisite knowledge and skills to assess, diagnose, and intervene in the event of complications or undesired outcomes and to institute nursing interventions in compliance with orders (including standing orders) or institutional protocols or guidelines.

    f. Demonstrate skill in airway management resuscitation.

    g. Demonstrate knowledge of the legal ramifications of administering intravenous conscious sedation and/or monitoring patients receiving intravenous conscious sedation, including the RN's responsibility and liability in the event of an untoward reaction or life-threatening complication.

6. The institution or practice setting has in place an educational/competency validation mechanism that includes a process for evaluating and documenting the individuals' demonstration of the knowledge, skills, and abilities related to the management of patients receiving intravenous conscious sedation. Evaluation and documentation of competence occur on a periodic basis according to institutional policy.

ADDITIONAL GUIDELINES

1. Intravenous access must be continuously maintained in the patient receiving intravenous conscious sedation.

2. All patients receiving intravenous conscious sedation will be continuously monitored throughout the procedure as well as the recovery phase by physiologic measurements including, but not limited to, respiratory rate, oxygen saturation, blood pressure, cardiac rate and rhythm, and patient's level of consciousness.

3. Supplemental oxygen will be immediately available to all patients receiving intravenous conscious sedation and administered per order (including standing orders).

4. An emergency cart with a defibrillator must be immediately accessible to every location where intravenous conscious sedation is administered. Suction and a positive pressure breathing device, oxygen, and appropriate airways must be in each room where intravenous conscious sedation is administered.

5. Provisions must be in place for backup personnel who are experts in airway management, emergency intubation, and advanced cardiopulmonary resuscitation if complications arise.

Endorsed by:
    American Association of Critical-Care Nurses
    American Association of Neuroscience Nurses
    American Association of Nurse Anesthetists
    American Association of Spinal Cord Injury Nurses
    American Association of Occupational Health Nurses
    American Nephrology Nurses Association
    American Nurses Association
    American Radiological Nurses Association
    American Society of Pain Management Nurses
    American Society of Plastic and Reconstructive Surgical Nurses
    American Society of Post Anesthesia Nurses
    American Urological Association, Allied
    Association of Operating Room Nurses
    Association of Pediatric Oncology Nurses
    Association of Rehabilitation Nurses
    Dermatology Nurses Association
    NAACOG, The Organization for Obstetric, Gynecologic, and Neonatal Nurses
    National Association of Orthopaedic Nurses
    National Flight Nurses Association
    National Student Nurses Association
    Nurse Consultants Association, Inc.
    Nurses Organization of Veterans Affairs
    Nursing Pain Association

American Association of Nurse Anesthetists Position Statement: Qualified Providers of Conscious Sedation*

POSITION

The American Association of Nurse Anesthetists (AANA) requires the safe administration of conscious sedation requires the sole attention of a professional who is educated in the specialty of anesthesia and skilled in the administration of conscious sedation, monitored anesthesia care, and regional and/or general anesthesia.

PURPOSE

The purpose of this statement is to provide guidance that will improve the quality of patient care when conscious sedation is administered.

BACKGROUND

Conscious sedation easily may be converted into deep sedation and/or loss of consciousness because of the unique characteristics of the drugs used as well as the physical status and drug sensitivities of the individual patient. The administration of conscious sedation requires constant monitoring of the patient and the ability to respond immediately to any deviation from normal. Conscious sedation should only be provided by an individual who is qualified to select and administer the appropriate drugs and who is capable of managing all anesthetic levels and potential complications, including airway management, intubation, and resuscitation. Appropriate monitoring devices, emergency drugs and equipment, and essential airway support equipment should be immediately available.

Although the AANA believes that optimal care for the patient receiving intravenous conscious sedation is best provided by a qualified anesthesia provider, the association also recognizes the reality of the increased demand for this service, which the current supply of anesthesia providers is unable to fully meet. In recent years, registered professional nurses in selected specialty areas of practice have become increasingly involved in assisting physicians in providing intravenous conscious sedation. Questions have been raised by nursing organizations and healthcare institutions concerning the appropriateness, nursing preparation, and patient/procedural requirements for this practice. In an effort to answer some of the concerns and to promote safe care during intravenous conscious sedation, the AANA has developed suggested guidelines for registered professional nurses who are involved in this patient care activity. (See Addendum: Suggested Guidelines for Registered Professional Nurses Engaged in the Administration of Intravenous Conscious Sedation.) These suggested guidelines do not supersede or consider the effect of more restrictive relevant laws, regulations, judicial and administrative decisions and interpretations, accepted standards and scopes of practice established by professional nursing organizations, and institutional policies applicable to registered professional nurses, which should be reviewed.

ADDENDUM TO POSITION STATEMENT 2.2: SUGGESTED GUIDELINES FOR REGISTERED PROFESSIONAL NURSES ENGAGED IN THE ADMINISTRATION OF INTRAVENOUS CONSCIOUS SEDATION

Preamble

Although optimal care for the patient receiving intravenous conscious sedation is best provided by a qualified anesthesia provider, the increased number of surgical and diagnostic procedures being performed and the growth in the number of practice settings in which intravenous conscious sedation is provided have created a demand that the current supply of anesthesia providers is unable to meet. In recent years, registered professional nurses in selected specialty areas of practice have become increasingly involved in assisting physicians in providing intravenous conscious sedation. In an effort to promote safe care during intravenous conscious sedation, to address questions which have been raised by nursing organizations and healthcare institutions with respect to the qualifications of registered professional nurses involved in this care, and taking into consideration the patient and procedural requirements for this practice, these suggested guidelines have been developed. These suggested guidelines do not supersede or consider the effect of more restrictive relevant laws, regulations, judicial and administrative decisions and interpretations, accepted standards and scopes of practice established by professional nursing organizations, and institutional policies applicable to registered professional nurses, which should be reviewed. A registered professional nurse engaged in intravenous conscious sedation may want to make certain that insurance coverage applies to these activities.

Introduction

Conscious sedation is defined as a minimally depressed level of consciousness that retains the patient's ability to maintain a patent airway independently and continuously and to respond appropriately to physical stimulation and/or verbal command.

Conscious sedation easily may be converted into deep sedation and/or loss of consciousness because of the unique characteristics of the drugs used as well as the physical status and drug sensitivities of the individual patient. The administration of conscious sedation requires constant monitoring of the patient and the ability to respond immediately to any deviation from normal. Vigilance of the provider and the ability to recognize and intervene in the event complications or undesired outcomes arise are essential requirements for individuals administering conscious sedation.

Suggested Guidelines

The following suggested guidelines require that registered professional nurses administering intravenous conscious sedation have (1) the requisite knowledge and skills, (2) resuscitation equipment and emergency drugs readily available, and (3) adequate back-up of expert emergency support personnel in the event complications arise.

First, management of intravenous conscious sedation during therapeutic, diagnostic, or surgical procedures by a registered professional nurse must be done in compliance with patient-specific written orders and may be performed by a registered professional nurse provided the following criteria are met:

1. Guidelines for patient monitoring, drug administration, and protocols for dealing with potential complications or emergency situations are available and have been developed in accordance with accepted standards of anesthesia practice.
2. The registered professional nurse managing the care of the patient receiving intravenous conscious sedation shall have no other responsibilities during the procedure and may not leave the patient unattended or engage in tasks that would compromise conscious monitoring.
3. A qualified professional capable of managing complications which might arise should remain on site until the patient is stable.
4. A qualified professional authorized to discharge a patient under institutional guidelines remains on site to discharge the patient in accordance with established criteria of the facility.

Second, to be qualified, the registered professional nurse managing the care of patients receiving intravenous conscious sedation must be able to:

1. Demonstrate the acquired knowledge of anatomy, physiology, pharmacology, cardiac arrhythmia recognition, and complications related to intravenous conscious sedation and medications.
2. Assess the total patient care requirement during intravenous conscious sedation. Physiologic measurements should include, but not be limited to, respiratory rate, oxygen saturation, blood pressure, cardiac rate and rhythm, and patient's level of consciousness. Documentation intervals should be dictated by the patient's condition; however, vital signs should be recorded at least every 5 minutes.

3. Understand the principles of oxygen delivery, transport and uptake, and respiratory physiology and understand and be able to use oxygen delivery devices.

4. Anticipate and recognize potential complications of intravenous conscious sedation in relation to the type of medication being administered.

5. Possess the requisite knowledge and skills to assess, diagnose, and intervene in the event of complications or undesired outcomes and to institute nursing interventions in compliance with orders (including standing orders) or institutional protocols or guidelines.

6. Demonstrate skill in airway management and resuscitation.

7. Have a thorough understanding and recognition of the legal ramifications of providing this care, especially of the responsibility and liability in the event of an untoward reaction or life-threatening complication.

Each institution or practice setting should have in place an educational/credentialing mechanism which includes a process for evaluating and documenting the individual's demonstration of the knowledge, skills, and abilities related to the management of patients receiving intravenous conscious sedation. Evaluation and documentation of competence should occur on a periodic basis.

The following procedural guidelines, which address monitoring modalities, emergency drugs and equipment, and ventilatory support personnel, should be incorporated into the institution's or healthcare facility's policies and procedures for the administration of intravenous conscious sedation:

1. All patients having local anesthesia with intravenous conscious sedation will have a continuous intravenous line in place.

2. All patients receiving intravenous conscious sedation will be continuously monitored throughout the procedure as well as the recovery phase by electrocardiogram, pulse oximetry, and blood pressure monitors.

3. Supplemental oxygen will be provided to all patients receiving intravenous conscious sedation per order (including standing orders).

4. An emergency cart must be immediately accessible to every location where intravenous conscious sedation is administered. This cart must include at least the following: emergency and resuscitative drugs, airway and ventilatory adjunct equipment, defibrillator, and a source for administration of 100% oxygen. A positive pressure breathing device, oxygen, and appropriate airways must be in each room where intravenous conscious sedation is administered.

5. Provisions must be in place for back-up personnel who are expert in airway management, emergency intubation, and advanced cardiopulmonary resuscitation if complications arise.

6. Registered professional nurses who are not credentialed anesthesia providers should not administer drugs classified as anesthetics, including but not limited to ketamine, sodium thiopental, methohexital, propofol, etomidate, and nitrous oxide.

BIBLIOGRAPHY

Applegeet, C.J. (1989). Perioperative nurse must constantly acquire new skills. *AORN Journal 50,* 950.

Bell, G.D., Bowen, S., Morden, A., et al. (1987). Prevention of hypoxaemia during upper gastrointestinal endoscopy by means of oxygen via nasal cannulae. *Lancet 1,* 1033.

Finnie, G. (1990). Conscious sedation and plastic surgery. *Specialty Nursing Forum 2,* 8.

Fogg, D.M. (1989). Recommendation for instrument counts: Testing sterilizers with biological indicators: Organizational structure of OR. *AORN Journal 49,* 1667.

Guidelines for the elective use of conscious sedation, deep sedation, and general anesthesia in pediatric patients. (1985). *Pediatrics 76,* 317.

Gunn, I.P. (1990). The many issues regarding IV conscious sedation. *Specialty Nursing Forum 2,* 2.

Harvard minimal monitoring standards. (1986). *Journal of the American Medical Association 256,* 8.

Kallar, S.K. (1991). Conscious sedation for outpatient surgery. *Wellcome Trends in Anesthesiology 9,* 8.

Kingsbury, J.A. (1990). IV conscious sedation: JCAHO and hospital issues. *Specialty Nursing Forum 2,* 7.

McDonald, J.S., et al. (1990). A second-time study of the anesthetist's intraoperative period. *British Journal of Anaesthesiology 64,* 582.

Murphy, E.K. (1988). Legal considerations in RN monitoring of intravenous sedation. *AORN Journal 48,* 1184.

Needleman, H.L. Conscious sedation for pediatric outpatient dental procedures. *International Anesthesiology Clinics 27,* 102.

Newman, P.W. (1990). IV conscious sedation: Nursing issues. *Specialty Nursing Forum 2,* 1, 4.

Petrone, S. (1989). Perioperative nurses must prepare themselves to monitor patients receiving local anesthesia. *AORN Journal 50,* 442.

Recommended practice: Monitoring the patient receiving local anesthesia. (1989). *AORN Journal 50,* 624.

Ryder, W., Wright, P.A. (1988). Dental sedation: A review. *British Dental Journal 165,* 207.

Separation of operator-anesthetist responsibilities. *American Association of Nurse Anesthetists Position Statement.* Park Ridge, IL, 1988.

Spry, C.C. (1990). Perioperative nurses should keep monitoring within their specialty. *AORN Journal 51,* 1071.

Tucker, M.R., Ochs, M.W., White, R.P., Jr. (1986). Arterial blood gas levels after midazolam or diazepam administered with or without fentanyl as an intravenous sedative for outpatient surgical procedures. *Journal of Oral and Maxillofacial Surgery 44,* 688.

U.S. Department of Health and Human Services Office of Medical Applications of Research (1985). *Anesthesia and sedation in the dental office.* National Institutes of Health (NIH Consensus Development Conference Statement 5:10), Bethesda, MD.

Watson, D.S. (1990). Recommended practices for monitoring and administering IV conscious sedation. *Specialty Nursing Forum 2,* 3.

Watson, D.S., James, D.S. (1990). IV conscious sedation: Implications of monitoring patients receiving local anesthesia. *AORN Journal 51,* 1512.

American Society of Anesthesiologists Practice Guidelines for Sedation and Analgesia by Non-Anesthesiologists*

INTRODUCTION

Anesthesiologists possess specific expertise in the pharmacology, physiology, and clinical management of patients receiving sedation and analgesia. For this reason, they are frequently called upon to participate in the development of institutional policies and procedures for sedation and analgesia in non-operating-room settings. To assist in this process, the American Society of Anesthesiologists has developed these *Guidelines for Sedation and Analgesia by Non-Anesthesiologists.*

Practice guidelines are systematically developed recommendations that assist practitioners in making decisions about health care. These recommendations may be adopted, modified, exceeded, or rejected according to clinical needs and constraints, and they are subject to periodic revision as warranted by the evolution of medical knowledge, technology, and practice. Practice guidelines are not intended as standards or absolute requirements, and their use cannot guarantee any specific outcome.

The practice guidelines enumerated below have been developed using systematic literature summarization techniques. Results of the literature analyses have been supplemented by the opinions of the Task Force members and a panel of more than 60 consultants, drawn from a variety of medical specialties where sedation and analgesia are commonly provided. In those instances where the literature does not provide conclusive data, there is an explicit statement that the guidelines are based on the opinion of the consultants or the consensus of the Task Force members. A detailed description of the analytic methods is included in Appendix 1 (see p. 237).

DEFINITION

"Sedation and analgesia" describes a state which allows patients to tolerate unpleasant procedures while maintaining adequate cardiorespiratory function and the

---

*Reprinted with the permission of the Association of Anesthesiologists Task Force on Sedation and Analgesia by Non-Anesthesiologists and Lippincott-Raven.
Task Force on Sedation and Analgesia by Non-Anesthesiologists: Jeffrey B. Gross, MD, Chair; Peter L. Bailey, MD; Charles J. Coté, MD; Fred G. Davis, MD; Burton S. Epstein, MD; Patricia A. Kapur, MD; John M. Zerwas, MD; Gregory Zuccaro, Jr., MD; Richard T. Connis, PhD, Methodologist

ability to respond purposefully to verbal command and/or tactile stimulation. The Task Force decided that the term "sedation and analgesia" (sedation/analgesia) more accurately defines this therapeutic goal than does the commonly used but imprecise term "conscious sedation." Note that patients whose only response is reflex withdrawal from a painful stimulus are sedated to a greater degree than encompassed by "sedation/analgesia."

PURPOSE

The purpose of these guidelines is to allow clinicians to provide their patients with the benefits of sedation/analgesia while minimizing the associated risks. Sedation/analgesia provides two general types of benefit. First, sedation/analgesia allows patients to tolerate unpleasant procedures by relieving anxiety, discomfort, or pain. Second, in children and uncooperative adults, sedation/analgesia may expedite the conduct of procedures which are not particularly uncomfortable but which require that the patient not move. Excessive sedation/analgesia may result in cardiac or respiratory depression which must be rapidly recognized and appropriately managed to avoid the risk of hypoxic brain damage, cardiac arrest, or death. Conversely, inadequate sedation/analgesia may result in undue patient discomfort or actual patient injury because of lack of cooperation or adverse physiological response to stress.

FOCUS

These guidelines have been designed to be applicable to procedures performed in a variety of settings (e.g., hospitals, free-standing clinics, physicians' offices) by practitioners who are not specialists in anesthesiology. The guidelines specifically exclude the following: (1) patients who are not undergoing a diagnostic or therapeutic procedure (e.g., post-operative analgesia, sedation for treatment of insomnia); (2) otherwise healthy patients receiving peripheral nerve blocks, local or topical anesthesia, or no more than 50% N_2O with O_2 with no other sedative or analgesic agents administered by any route; (3) situations where it is anticipated that the required sedation will eradicate the purposeful response to verbal commands or tactile stimulation (as distinct from reflex withdrawal from a painful stimulus); such patients require a greater level of care than recommended by these guidelines; and (4) perioperative management of patients undergoing general anesthesia or major conduction anesthesia (spinal or epidural/caudal blockade).

APPLICATION

These guidelines are intended to be general in their application and broad in scope. The appropriate choice of agents and techniques for sedation/analgesia is dependent upon the experience and preference of the individual practitioner, requirements or constraints imposed by the patient or procedure, and the likelihood of producing unintended loss of consciousness. Templates are provided as examples to illustrate principles; clinicians and their institutions have ultimate responsibility for selecting patients, procedures, medications, and equipment.

GUIDELINES

PATIENT EVALUATION

Published data suggest and consultant opinion strongly supports the contention that appropriate pre-procedure evaluation of patients' histories and physical findings reduces the risk of adverse outcomes. Additionally, consultant opinion supports the contention that an appropriate history, physical examination, and laboratory evaluation leads to improved patient satisfaction.

Recommendations. Clinicians administering sedation/analgesia should be familiar with relevant aspects of the patient's medical history, including (1) abnormalities of the major organ systems, (2) previous adverse experience with sedation/analgesia and regional and general anesthesia, (3) current medications and drug allergies, (4) time and nature of last oral intake, and (5) history of tobacco, alcohol, or substance use or abuse. Patients presenting for sedation/analgesia should undergo a focused physical examination including auscultation of the heart and lungs and evaluation of the airway (see Template 1, p. 234). Pre-procedure laboratory testing should be guided by the patient's underlying medical condition and the likelihood that the results will affect the management of sedation/analgesia.

PRE-PROCEDURE PREPARATION

Patient Counseling

There is insufficient evidence in the literature to establish the benefit of providing the patient (or his/her guardian, in the case of a child or impaired adult) with pre-procedure information about sedation/analgesia. However, the consultants strongly support the contention that appropriate pre-procedure counseling improves patient satisfaction and reduces risks; they also support the view that costs may be reduced. The Task Force members concur that patients undergoing sedation/analgesia should be informed of the benefits, risks, and limitations associated with this therapy, as well as possible alternatives.

Pre-Procedure Fasting

Because sedatives and analgesics tend to impair airway reflexes in proportion to the degree of sedation/analgesia achieved, members of the Task Force support the concept of pre-procedure fasting prior to sedation/analgesia for elective procedures. However, the literature provides insufficient data to test the hypothesis that pre-procedure fasting results in a decreased incidence of adverse outcomes in patients undergoing sedation/analgesia (as distinct from patients undergoing general anesthesia).

Recommendations. Patients (or their legal guardians in the case of minors or legally incompetent adults) should be informed of and agree to the administration of sedation/analgesia before the procedure begins. Patients undergoing sedation/analgesia for elective procedures should not drink fluids or eat solid foods for a sufficient period of time to allow for gastric emptying prior to their procedure (see Template 2, p. 234). In urgent, emergent, or other situations where gastric emptying is impaired, the potential for pulmonary aspiration of gastric contents must be considered in determining the timing of the intervention and the degree of sedation/analgesia.

MONITORING
Level of Consciousness
The response of patients to commands during procedures performed with sedation/analgesia serves as a guide to their level of consciousness. Spoken responses also provide an indication that the patients are breathing. Patients whose only response is reflex withdrawal from painful stimuli are likely to be deeply sedated, approaching a state of general anesthesia, and should be treated accordingly. The consultants strongly support the contention that monitoring level consciousness reduces risks, and support the concept that overall costs may be reduced as well. The members of the Task Force believe that many of the complications associated with sedation/analgesia can be avoided if adverse drug responses are detected and treated in a timely manner (i.e., prior to the development of cardiovascular decompensation or cerebral hypoxia); this may pose a special risk to patients given sedatives/analgesics in unmonitored settings in anticipation of a subsequent procedure.

Pulmonary Ventilation
It is the opinion of the Task Force that a primary cause of morbidity associated with sedation/analgesia is drug-induced respiratory depression. The literature suggests and consultant opinion strongly supports the observation that monitoring of ventilatory function reduces the risk of adverse outcomes associated with sedation/analgesia. Ventilatory function can usually be effectively monitored by observation of spontaneous respiratory activity or auscultation of breath sounds. In circumstances where patients are physically separated from the care giver, the consultants support and the Task Force members concur that automated apnea monitoring (by detection of exhaled CO_2 or other means) may decrease risks; the consultants suggest that such monitoring will *not* reduce overall costs. The Task Force cautions practitioners that impedance plethysmography may fail to detect airway obstruction.

Oxygenation

Published data suggest and the consultants strongly support the view that early detection of hypoxemia through the use of oximetry during sedation/analgesia decreases the likelihood of adverse outcomes such as cardiac arrest and death. The literature suggests, the consultants strongly support, and Task Force members agree that hypoxemia during sedation and analgesia is more likely to be detected by oximetry than by clinical assessment alone. The Task Force emphasizes that oximetry is not a substitute for monitoring ventilatory function.

Hemodynamics

Although there is insufficient published data to reach a conclusion, it is the opinion of the Task Force that sedative and analgesic agents may blunt the appropriate autonomic compensation for hypovolemia and procedure-related stresses. Early detection of changes in patients' heart rate and blood pressure may enable practitioners to detect problems and intervene in a timely fashion, reducing the risk of cardiovascular collapse. The consultants support the concept that regular monitoring of vital signs reduces risks and suggest that it decreases costs as well. Although the literature provides no guidance, the consultants suggest the use of continuous electrocardiographic monitoring in patients with hypertension and strongly support its use in patients with significant cardiovascular disease or dysrhythmias; the consultants suggest that electrocardiographic monitoring is not required in patients without cardiovascular disease.

Recommendations. Monitoring of patient response to verbal commands should be routine, except in patients who are unable to respond appropriately (e.g., young children, mentally impaired or uncooperative patients) or during procedures where facial movement could be detrimental. During procedures where a verbal response is not possible (e.g., oral surgery, upper endoscopy), the ability to give a "thumbs up" or other indication of consciousness in response to verbal or tactile (light tap) stimulation suggests that the patient will be able to control his airway and take deep breaths if necessary. Note that a response limited to reflex withdrawal from a painful stimulus represents a greater degree of sedation/analgesia than addressed by this document.

Ventilatory function should be continually monitored by observation and/or auscultation. When ventilation cannot be directly observed, exhaled CO_2 detection is a useful adjunct to these modalities. All patients undergoing sedation/analgesia should be monitored by pulse oximetry with appropriate alarms. If available, the variable-pitch "beep," which gives a continuous audible indication of the oxygen saturation reading, may be helpful. When possible, blood pressure should be determined before sedation/analgesia is initiated. Once sedation/analgesia is established, blood pressure should be measured at regular intervals during the procedure, as well as during the recovery period. Electrocardiographic monitoring should be used in patients with significant cardiovascular disease as well as during procedures where dysrhythmias are anticipated.

RECORDING OF MONITORED PARAMETERS

Both the literature and consultant opinion suggest that contemporaneous recording of patients' level of consciousness, respiratory function, and hemodynamics reduces the risk of adverse outcomes. While consultant opinion suggests that recording of this information may not improve patient comfort or satisfaction, the consultants suggest that it may reduce costs resulting from adverse events. The consultants strongly support recording of vital signs and respiratory variables before initiating sedation/analgesia, after administration of sedative/analgesic medications, at regular intervals during the procedure, upon initiation of recovery, and immediately before discharge. It is the opinion of the Task Force that contemporaneous recording (either automatic or manual) of patient data provides information which could prove critical in determining the cause of any adverse events which might occur. Additionally, manual recording ensures that an individual caring for the patient is aware of changes in patient status in a timely fashion.

Recommendations. Patients' ventilatory and oxygenation status and hemodynamic variables should be recorded at a frequency to be determined by the type and amount of medication administered as well as the length of the procedure and the general condition of the patient. At a minimum, this should be (1) before the beginning of the procedure, (2) following the administration of sedative/analgesic agents, (3) upon completion of the procedure, (4) during initial recovery, and (5) at the time of discharge. If recording is performed automatically, device alarms should be set to alert the care team to critical changes in patient status.

AVAILABILITY OF A STAFF PERSON DEDICATED <u>SOLELY</u> TO PATIENT MONITORING AND SAFETY

Although there are insufficient data in the literature to provide guidance on this issue, the Task Force recognizes that it is difficult for the individual performing a procedure to be fully cognizant of the patient's condition during sedation/analgesia. The consultants support the contention that the availability of an individual other than the person performing the procedure to monitor the patient's status improves patient comfort and satisfaction; they also strongly support the view that risks are reduced. The consultants support the observation that this would not decrease overall costs. It is the consensus of the Task Force members that the individual monitoring the patient may assist the practitioner with interruptible ancillary tasks of short duration once the patient's level of sedation/analgesia and vital signs have stabilized, provided that adequate monitoring is maintained.

Recommendation. A designated individual, other than the practitioner performing the procedure, should be present to monitor the patient throughout procedures performed with sedation/analgesia. This individual may assist with minor interruptible tasks.

TRAINING OF PERSONNEL

Although there is insufficient literature to determine the effectiveness of training on patient outcomes, the consultants strongly support the observation that providing appropriate training in clinical pharmacology for individuals administering sedative/analgesic medications reduces the risk of adverse outcomes; they also support the view that patient comfort is improved and overall costs are reduced. Specific concerns include (1) potentiation of sedative-induced respiratory depression by concomitantly administered opioids, (2) inadequate time intervals between doses of sedative or analgesic agents resulting in cumulative overdose, and (3) inadequate familiarity with the role of pharmacologic antagonists for sedative and analgesic agents.

Because the primary complications of sedation/analgesia are related to respiratory or cardiovascular depression, it is the consensus of the Task Force that the individual responsible for monitoring the patient should be trained in the recognition of complications associated with sedation/analgesia. In addition, at least one qualified individual, capable of establishing a patent airway and maintaining ventilation and oxygenation, should be present during the procedure.

Recommendations. Individuals responsible for patients receiving sedation/analgesia should understand the pharmacology of the agents that are administered, as well as the role of pharmacologic antagonists for opioids and benzodiazepines. Individuals monitoring patients receiving sedation/analgesia should be able to recognize the associated complications. At least one individual capable of establishing a patent airway and positive pressure ventilation, as well as a means of summoning additional assistance, should be present whenever sedation/analgesia are administered. It is recommended that an individual with advanced life support skills be immediately available.

AVAILABILITY OF EMERGENCY EQUIPMENT

The literature suggests and the consultants strongly support the view that the ready availability of appropriately-sized emergency equipment reduces the risk of sedation and analgesia. The consultants also support the contention that overall costs, including those associated with adverse outcomes, may be reduced. The literature does not address the need for cardiac defibrillators during sedation/analgesia. The consultants strongly support the availability of a defibrillator whenever sedation/analgesia are administered.

Recommendations. Pharmacologic antagonists as well as appropriately sized equipment for establishing a patent airway and providing positive pressure ventilation with supplemental oxygen should be present whenever sedation/analgesia is administered. Advanced airway equipment and resuscitation medications should be immediately available (e.g., Template 3, p. 235). A defibrillator should be immediately available when sedation/analgesia is administered to patients with significant cardiovascular disease.

USE OF SUPPLEMENTAL OXYGEN

The literature supports the use of supplemental oxygen during sedation/analgesia. There is a decreased incidence and severeness of hypoxemia among sedation/analgesia patients given oxygen as compared to those breathing room air. However, it must be appreciated that by delaying the onset of hypoxemia supplemental oxygen will delay the detection of apnea by pulse oximetry, emphasizing the importance of monitoring pulmonary ventilation by other means (see above). Consultant opinion supports the view that supplemental oxygen decreases patient risk, while suggesting that routine use of supplemental oxygen may increase costs.

Recommendations. Equipment to administer supplemental oxygen should be present when sedation/analgesia is administered. If hypoxemia is anticipated or develops during sedation/analgesia, supplemental oxygen should be administered.

USE OF MULTIPLE SEDATIVE/ANALGESIC AGENTS

The literature supports the observation that combinations of agents may be more effective than single agents in certain circumstances. However, the published data also suggest and consultant opinion supports the observation that combinations of sedatives and opioids may increase the likelihood of adverse outcomes, including ventilatory depression and hypoxemia. Although not evaluated in the literature, it is the consensus of the Task Force that fixed combinations of sedative and analgesic agents may not allow the individual components of sedation/analgesia to be appropriately titrated to meet the individual requirements of the patient and procedure.

Recommendations. Combinations of sedative and analgesic agents should be administered as appropriate for the procedure being performed and the condition of the patient. Ideally, each component should be administered individually to achieve the desired effect (e.g., additional analgesic medication to relieve pain, additional sedative medication to decrease awareness or anxiety). The propensity for combinations of sedative and analgesic agents to potentiate respiratory depression emphasizes the need to appropriately reduce the dose of each component as well as the need to continually monitor respiratory function.

TITRATION OF SEDATIVE/ANALGESIC MEDICATIONS TO ACHIEVE THE DESIRED EFFECT

The literature suggests that the administration of small incremental doses of intravenous sedative/analgesic drugs until the desired level of sedation and/or analgesia is achieved is preferable to a single dose based on patient size, weight, or age. The consultants support the concept that incremental drug administration improves patient comfort and decreases costs; they strongly support the contention that the potential risks associated with excessive doses are reduced.

Recommendations. Intravenous sedative/analgesic drugs should be given in small incremental doses which are titrated to the desired endpoints of analgesia and sedation. Sufficient time must elapse between doses to allow the effect of each dose to be assessed before subsequent drug administration. When drugs are administered by non-intravenous routes (e.g., oral, rectal, intramuscular), allowance should be made for the time required for drug absorption before supplementation is considered.

INTRAVENOUS ACCESS

Published data suggest that in cooperative patients administration of sedative/ analgesic agents by the intravenous route improves patient comfort and satisfaction. The consultants strongly support the importance of intravenous access in reducing patient risks. In situations where sedative/analgesic medications are to be administered intravenously, it is the consensus of the Task Force that maintaining intravenous access until the patient is no longer at risk for cardiorespiratory depression improves patient safety. In those situations where sedation is begun by non-intravenous routes (e.g., oral, rectal, intramuscular) the need for intravenous access is not sufficiently addressed in the literature. However, initiation of intravenous access after the initial sedation takes effect allows additional sedative/analgesic and resuscitation drugs to be administered if necessary.

Recommendations. In patients receiving intravenous medications for sedation/analgesia, vascular access should be maintained throughout the procedure and until the patient is no longer at risk for cardiorespiratory depression. In patients who have received sedation/analgesia by non-intravenous routes, or whose intravenous line has become dislodged or blocked, practitioners should determine the advisability of establishing or reestablishing intravenous access on a case-by-case basis. In all instances, an individual with the skills to establish intravenous access should be immediately available.

REVERSAL AGENTS

Specific antagonist agents are available for the opioids (e.g., naloxone) and benzodiazepines (e.g., flumazenil). The literature supports the ability of naloxone to reverse opioid-induced sedation and ventilatory depression during sedation/analgesia. However, the Task Force reminds practitioners that acute reversal of opioid-induced analgesia may result in pain, hypertension, tachycardia, or pulmonary edema. The literature supports the ability of flumazenil to reverse benzodiazepine-induced sedation and its effectiveness in reversing ventilatory depression in patients who have received benzodiazepines alone. In patients who have received both benzodiazepines and opioids, published data support the ability of flumazenil to reverse sedation; however, there are insufficient data to establish the effectiveness of flumazenil in reversing ventilatory depression under these circumstances. The consultants strongly support the contention that the availability of reversal agents is associated with decreased risk. It is the consensus of the Task Force that respiratory depression should be initially treated with supplemental oxygen and, if necessary, positive pressure ventilation by mask.

Recommendations. Specific antagonists should be available whenever opioid analgesics or benzodiazepines are administered for sedation/analgesia. Naloxone and/or flumazenil may be administered to improve spontaneous ventilatory efforts in patients who have received opioids or benzodiazepines, respectively. This may be especially helpful in cases where airway control and positive pressure ventilation are difficult. Prior to or concomitantly with pharmacological reversal, patients who become hypoxemic or apneic during sedation/analgesia should (1) be encouraged or stimulated to breathe deeply, (2) receive positive pressure ventilation if spontaneous ventilation is inadequate, and (3) receive supplemental oxygen. Following pharmacological reversal, patients should be observed long enough to ensure that cardiorespiratory depression does not recur.

RECOVERY CARE

Patients may continue to be at significant risk for developing complications after their procedure is completed. Decreased procedural stimulation, prolonged drug absorption following oral or rectal administration, and post-procedure hemorrhage may contribute to cardiorespiratory depression. When sedation/analgesia is administered to outpatients, one must assume that there will be no medical supervision once the patient leaves the medical facility. Although there is not sufficient literature to examine the effects of post-procedure monitoring on patient outcomes, the consultants suggest that appropriate monitoring of patients during the recovery period will improve patient comfort and strongly support the view that adverse outcomes may be reduced. It is the consensus of the Task Force that discharge criteria should be established which minimize the risk for cardiorespiratory depression after patients are released from observation by trained personnel.

Recommendations. Following sedation/analgesia, patients should be observed until they are no longer at increased risk for cardiorespiratory depression. Vital signs and respiratory function should be monitored at regular intervals until patients are suitable for discharge. Discharge criteria should be designed to minimize the risk of central nervous system or cardiorespiratory depression following discharge from observation by trained personnel (see Template 4, p. 236).

SPECIAL SITUATIONS

The literature suggests, the consultants strongly support, and the task force members concur that certain classes of patients (e.g., uncooperative patients; extremes of age;

severe cardiac, pulmonary, hepatic, renal, or central nervous system disease; morbid obesity; sleep apnea; pregnancy; drug or alcohol abuse) are at increased risk for developing complications related to sedation/analgesia unless special precautions are taken. However, the consultants support the view that risks may be reduced by pre-procedure consultation with appropriate specialists (e.g., cardiologist, pulmonologist, nephrologist, obstetrician, pediatrician, anesthesiologist) before administration of sedation/analgesia to these individuals. The consultants support the concept that patient comfort is improved and risks are reduced by consultation with an anesthesiologist before administering sedation/analgesia to patients who are likely to develop complications (e.g., inadequate spontaneous ventilation, loss of airway control, cardiovascular compromise) or in whom sedation/analgesia alone is not expected to provide adequate conditions (e.g., young children, uncooperative patients). However, the consultants also support the contention that such consultation will not reduce costs.

Recommendations. Whenever possible, appropriate medical specialists should be consulted prior to administration of sedation/analgesia to patients with significant underlying conditions. The choice of specialists depends on the nature of the underlying condition and the urgency of the situation. For significantly compromised patients (e.g., severe obstructive pulmonary disease, coronary artery disease, or congestive heart failure), or if it appears likely that sedation to the point of unresponsiveness or general anesthesia will be necessary to obtain adequate conditions, practitioners who are not specifically qualified to provide these modalities should consult an anesthesiologist.

TEMPLATE 1	*Example of Airway Assessment Procedures for Sedation and Analgesia*

Positive pressure ventilation, with or without endotracheal intubation, may be necessary if respiratory compromise develops during sedation/analgesia. This may be more difficult in patients with atypical airway anatomy. Also, some airway abnormalities may increase the likelihood of airway obstruction during spontaneous ventilation. Some factors which may be associated with difficulty in airway management are:

HISTORY

Previous problems with anesthesia or sedation
Stridor, snoring, or sleep apnea
Dysmorphic facial features (e.g., Pierre-Robin syndrome, trisomy 21)
Advanced rheumatoid arthritis

PHYSICAL EXAMINATION

Habitus:	Significant obesity (especially involving the neck and facial structures)
Head and neck:	Short neck, limited neck extension, decreased hyoid-mental distance (<3 cm in an adult), neck mass, cervical spine disease or trauma, tracheal deviation
Mouth:	Small opening (<3 cm in an adult); edentulous; protruding incisors; loose or capped teeth; high, arched palate; macroglossia; tonsillar hypertrophy; non-visible uvula
Jaw:	Micrognathia, retrognathia, trismus, significant malocclusion

TEMPLATE 2	*Example of Fasting Protocol for Sedation and Analgesia for Elective Procedures*

Gastric emptying may be influenced by many factors, including anxiety, pain, abnormal autonomic function (e.g., diabetes), pregnancy, and mechanical obstruction. Therefore, the suggestions below do not guarantee that complete gastric emptying has occurred. Unless contraindicated, pediatric patients should be offered clear liquids until 2 to 3 hours before sedation to minimize the risk of dehydration.

	Solids and Nonclear Liquids*	Clear Liquids
Adults	6-8 hours or none after midnight†	2-3 hours
Children >36 months old	6-8 hours	2-3 hours
Children 6-36 months old	6 hours	2-3 hours
Children <6 months old	4-6 hours	2 hours

*This includes milk, formula, and breast milk (high fat content may delay gastric emptying).
†There are no data to establish whether a 6-8 hour fast is equivalent to an overnight fast prior to sedation/analgesia.

TEMPLATE 3 — *Example of Emergency Equipment for Sedation and Analgesia*

Appropriate emergency equipment should be available whenever sedative or analgesic drugs, capable of causing cardiorespiratory depression, are administered. The information below should be used as a guide, which should be modified depending upon the individual practice circumstances. Items in brackets [ ] are recommended when infants or children are sedated.

INTRAVENOUS EQUIPMENT

Gloves

Tourniquets

Alcohol wipes

Sterile gauze pads

Intravenous catheters [24, 22 gauge]

Intravenous tubing [pediatric "microdrip" —60 drops/ml]

Intravenous fluid

Three-way stopcocks

Assorted needles for drug aspiration, intramuscular injection [intraosseous bone marrow needle]

Appropriately sized syringes

Tape

BASIC AIRWAY MANAGEMENT EQUIPMENT

Source of compressed O_2 (tank with regulator or pipeline supply with flowmeter)

Source of suction

Suction catheters [pediatric suction catheters]

Yankauer-type suction

Face masks [infant/child face masks]

Self-inflating breathing bag-valve set [pediatric bag-valve set]

Oral and nasal airways [infant/child sized airways]

Lubricant

ADVANCED AIRWAY MANAGEMENT EQUIPMENT (FOR PRACTITIONERS WITH INTUBATION SKILLS)

Laryngoscope handles (tested)

Laryngoscope blades [pediatric laryngoscope blades]

Endotracheal tubes:

- Cuffed 6.0, 7.0, 8.0 mm i.d.
- [Uncuffed 2.5, 3.0, 3.5, 4.0, 4.5, 5.0, 5.5, 6.0 mm i.d.]

Stylet [appropriately sized for endotracheal tubes]

PHARMACOLOGIC ANTAGONISTS

Naloxone

Flumazenil

EMERGENCY MEDICATIONS

Epinephrine

Ephedrine

Atropine

Lidocaine

Glucose (50%) [10% or 25% glucose]

Diphenhydramine

Hydrocortisone, methylprednisolone, or dexamethasone

Diazepam or midazolam

Ammonia spirits

TEMPLATE **4** *Example of Recovery and Discharge Criteria Following Sedation and Analgesia*

Each patient-care facility in which sedation/analgesia is administered should develop recovery and discharge criteria which are suitable for its specific patients and procedures. Some of the basic principles which might be incorporated in these criteria are enumerated below.

GENERAL PRINCIPLES

1. All patients receiving sedation/analgesia should be monitored until appropriate discharge criteria are satisfied. The duration of monitoring must be individualized depending upon the level of sedation achieved, the overall condition of the patient, and the nature of the intervention for which sedation/analgesia was administered.

2. The recovery area should be equipped with appropriate monitoring and resuscitation equipment.

3. A nurse or other trained individual should be in attendance until discharge criteria are fulfilled. An individual capable of establishing a patent airway and providing positive pressure ventilation should be immediately available.

4. Level of consciousness and vital signs (including frequency and depth of respiration in the absence of stimulation) should be recorded at regular intervals during recovery. The responsible practitioner should be notified if vital signs fall outside of the limits previously established for each patient.

GUIDELINES FOR DISCHARGE

1. Patients should be alert and oriented; infants and patients whose mental status was initially abnormal should have returned to their baseline. Practitioners must be aware that pediatric patients are at risk for airway obstruction should the head fall forward while the child is secured in a car seat.

2. Vital signs should be stable and within acceptable limits.

3. Sufficient time (up to 2 hours) should have elapsed following the last administration of reversal agents (naloxone, flumazenil) to ensure that patients do not become resedated after reversal effects have worn off.

4. Outpatients should be discharged in the presence of a responsible adult who will accompany them home and be able to report any post-procedure complications.

5. Outpatients should be provided with written instructions regarding post-procedure diet, medications, activities, and a phone number to be called in case of emergency.

APPENDIX 1: METHODS AND ANALYSES

The scientific assessment of these guidelines was based on the following statements, or evidence linkages. These linkages represent directional hypotheses about relationships between sedation/analgesia by non-anesthesiologists and clinical outcomes.

1. A pre-procedure patient evaluation (i.e., history, physical examination, laboratory evaluation) improves patient satisfaction, increases clinical benefits, and reduces adverse outcomes.
2. Pre-procedure preparation of the patient (e.g., counseling, fasting) improves patient satisfaction, increases clinical benefits, and reduces adverse outcomes.
3. Patient monitoring (i.e., level of consciousness, pulmonary ventilation, oxygenation, hemodynamics) improves patient satisfaction, increases clinical benefits, and reduces adverse outcomes.
4. Contemporaneous recording of monitored parameters (e.g., level of consciousness, respiratory function, hemodynamics) improves patient satisfaction, increases clinical benefits, and reduces adverse outcomes.
5. Availability of a staff person dedicated solely to patient monitoring and safety improves patient satisfaction, increases clinical benefits, and reduces adverse outcomes.
6. Education and training of [sedation/analgesia] providers improves patient satisfaction, increases clinical benefits, and reduces adverse outcomes.
7. Availability of appropriately sized emergency and airway equipment, including trained staff improves patient satisfaction, increases clinical benefits, and reduces adverse outcomes.
8. Use of supplemental oxygen improves patient satisfaction, increases clinical benefits, and reduces adverse outcomes.
9. Use of multiple sedative/analgesic agents improves patient satisfaction, increase clinical benefits, and reduces adverse outcomes.
10. Titration of sedative/analgesic medications to achieve the desired effect improves patient satisfaction, increases clinical benefits, and reduces adverse outcomes.
11. Administration of sedative/analgesic agents by the intravenous route improves patient satisfaction, increases clinical benefits, and reduces adverse outcomes.
12. Availability of reversal agents (e.g., naloxone, flumazenil) improves patient satisfaction, increases clinical benefits, and reduces adverse outcomes.
13. Postprocedure monitoring (e.g., during duration of recovery stay, post-discharge) improves patient satisfaction, increases clinical benefits, and reduces adverse outcomes.
14. Special regimens for patients with special problems (e.g., uncooperative patients, extremes of age, severe cardiac, pulmonary, hepatic, renal or CNS disease, morbid obesity, sleep apnea, pregnancy, drug or alcohol abuse, emergency/unprepared patients, metabolic and airway difficulties) improves patient satisfaction, increase clinical benefits, and reduce adverse outcomes.

Scientific evidence was derived from multiple sources, including aggregated research literature (with meta-analyses when appropriate), surveys, open presentations, and other consensus-oriented activities. For purposes of literature aggregation, potentially relevant clinical studies were identified via electronic and manual searches of the literature. The electronic search covered a 29-year period from 1966 to 1994. Manual searches covered a 48-year period from 1947 through 1994. Over 3000 citations were initially identified, yielding a total of 1315 non-overlapping articles that addressed topics related to the 14 evidence linkages. Following review of the articles, 1046 studies did not provide direct evidence and were subsequently eliminated, yielding a total of 269 articles containing direct linkage-related evidence. Journals represented by the 269 articles included the following disciplines: anesthesiology, 59; oncology, 5; cardiology, 12; oral/maxillofacial/dental, 71; emergency medicine, 19; gastroenterology, 50; lithotripsy, 4; obstetrics/gynecology, 5; pediatrics, 4; pharmacology, 7; pulmonary medicine, 4; radiology, 17; surgery, 8; urology, 4.

A directional result for each study was initially determined by classifying the outcome as either (1) supporting a linkage, (2) refuting a linkage, or (3) neutral. The results were then averaged to obtain a directional assessment of support for each linkage. The literature relating to linkages 8 (supplemental oxygen), 9 (multiple agents), and 12a, 12b, and 12c (naloxone to reverse opioids, flumazenil to reverse benzodiazepines, and flumazenil to reverse benzodiazepines combined with opioids, respectively) contained enough studies with well-defined experimental designs and statistical information to conduct formal meta-analyses. Combined probability tests were applied when studies reported continuous data, and an odds-ratio procedure was applied to dichotomous study results.

Two combined probability tests were employed as follows: (1) The Fisher combined test, producing chi-square values based on logarithmic transformations of the reported p values from the independent studies and (2) the Stouffer combined test, providing weighted representation of the studies by weighting each of the standard normal deviates by the size of the sample. A procedure based on the Mantel-Haenszel method for combining study results using 2×2 tables was used when sufficient outcome frequency information was available. An acceptable significance level was set at $p < 0.01$ (one-tailed) and effect size estimates were calculated. Interobserver agreement was established through assessment of interrater reliability testing. Tests for heterogeneity of the independent samples were conducted to assure consistency among the study results. To control for potential publishing bias, a "fail-safe N" value was calculated for each combined probability test. No search for unpublished studies was conducted, and no reliability tests for locating research results were done.

Results of the combined probability tests are reported in Table 1. Significance levels from the weighted Stouffer combined tests for clinical efficacy were $p < 0.001$ for four linkages: 9 (multiple agents), 12a (naloxone for opioid reversal), 12b (flumazenil for benzodiazepine reversal), and 12c (flumazenil for benzodiazepine-opioid combinations). Weighted effect size estimates ranged from $r = 0.20$ to $r =$

| TABLE | 1 | *Statistical Summary* |

COMBINED TEST RESULTS: SEDATION EFFICACY

Linkage #9: Multiple Agents

Fisher combined test:	χ^2 92.54, p < 0.001, df 38
Stouffer combined test:	Zc (weighted) 5.270, p < 0.001
Effect size estimate:	r (weighted) 0.20
Fail-safe N value:	Nfs 0.01 117.9

COMBINED TEST RESULTS: REVERSAL EFFICACY

Linkage #12a: Naloxone to Reverse Opioids

Fisher combined test:	χ^2 50.66, p < 0.001, df 10
Stouffer combined test:	Zc (weighted) 3.894, p < 0.001
Effect size estimate:	r (weighted) 0.36
Fail-safe N value:	Nfs 0.01 24.6

Linkage #12b: Flumazenil to Reverse Benzodiazepines

Fisher combined test:	χ^2 220.54, p < 0.001, df 46
Stouffer combined test:	Zc (weighted) 6.450, p < 0.001
Effect size estimate:	r (weighted) 0.32
Fail-safe N value:	Nfs 0.01 628.4

Linkage #12c: Flumazenil to Reverse Benzodiazepines + Opioids

Fisher combined test:	χ^2 80.39, p < 0.001, df 12
Stouffer combined test:	Zc (weighted) 3.183, p < 0.001
Effect size estimate:	r (weighted) 0.42
Fail-safe N value:	Nfs 0.01 79.4

COMBINED TEST RESULTS: ADVERSE OUTCOMES

Linkage #9: Multiple Agents

Fisher combined test:	χ^2 86.17, p < 0.001, df 28
Stouffer combined test:	Zc (weighted) 3.716, p < 0.001
Effect size estimate:	r (weighted) 0.32
Fail-safe N value:	Nfs 0.01 127.9

COMBINED TEST RESULTS: BENEFICIAL RESPIRATORY OUTCOMES

Linkage #8: Supplemental Oxygen

Fisher combined test:	χ^2 73.95, p < 0.001, df 14
Stouffer combined test:	Zc (weighted) 7.227, p < 0.001
Effect size estimate:	r (weighted) 0.30
Fail-safe N value:	Nfs 0.01 61.3

Continued

TABLE 1 *Statistical Summary—cont'd*

Linkage #12a: Naloxone to Reverse Opioids

Fisher combined test:	χ^2 45.94, p < 0.001, df 10
Stouffer combined test:	Zc (weighted) 4.487, p < 0.001
Effect size estimate:	r (weighted) 0.36
Fail-safe N value:	Nfs 0.01 24.7

Linkage #12: Flumazenil to Reverse Benzodiazepines

Fisher combined test:	χ^2 29.07, p < 0.001, df 10
Stouffer combined test:	Zc (weighted) 0.740, p < 0.010, df (NS)
Effect size estimate:	r (weighted) 0.35
Fail-safe N value:	Nfs 0.01 9.8

0.42, demonstrating small-to-moderate effect size estimates. Significance levels from the weighted Stouffer combined tests for beneficial outcomes were p < 0.001 for two linkages, 8 (supplemental oxygen) and 12a (naloxone). Significance levels for adverse outcomes (p < 0.001) were found for linkage 9 (multiple agents). Linkage 12b was not significant. Weighted effect size estimates ranged from $r = 0.30$ to $r = 0.36$. Sufficient data were available to conduct Mantel-Haenszel analyses for linkages 8 (supplemental oxygen) and 9 (multiple agents). Significant differences in the odds of hypoxemia (assessed by S_pO_2 levels) were found between patients breathing supplemental oxygen versus those breathing room air (odds ratio = 4.68; 99% confidence limits = 4.13 to 5.23; $Z = 6.51$; p < 0.001). The odds of an adverse outcome for multiple agents were found to be non-significant.

Tests for heterogeneity of statistical tests and effects size were non-significant in all cases (p > 0.01) except linkage 9 (multiple agents) and 12c (flumazenil to reverse benzodiazepines combined with opioids), indicating that the majority of pooled studies provided common estimates of significance and population effect sizes for the linkages. The two significant effect size estimates for heterogeneity may be due to a variety of factors (e.g., methodological differences among the various studies, dissimilar outcome measures or other mediating effects).

Agreement among Task Force members and two methodologists was established by interrater reliability testing. Agreement levels using a Kappa statistic for two-rater agreement pairs were as follows: (1) type of study design, κ = 0.69 to 0.95; (2) type of analysis, κ = 0.48 to 0.81; (3) evidence linkage assignment, κ = 0.65 to 0.90; and (4) literature inclusion for database, κ = 0.35 to 1.00. Three-rater chance-corrected agreement values were (1) design, S_{av} = 0.79, Var (S_{av}) = 0.06; (2) analysis, S_{av} = 0.61, Var (S_{av}) = 0.06; (3) linkage identification, S_{av} = 0.74, Var (S_{av}) = 0.01; (4) literature inclusion, S_{av} = 0.53, Var (S_{av}) = 0.02. These values represent moderate to high levels of agreement.

The findings of the literature analyses were supplemented by the opinions of Task Force members as well as by surveys of the opinions of a panel of consultants drawn from the following specialties where sedation/analgesia are commonly administered: anesthesiology, 9; cardiology, 5; dental anesthesiology, 3; dermatology, 1; emergency medicine, 3; gastroenterology, 6; hematology/oncology, 2; intensive care, 2; oral and maxillofacial surgery, 5; pediatric dentistry, 2; pediatric oncology, 1; pharmacology, 2; plastic surgery, 1; pulmonary medicine, 5; radiology, 8; surgery, 4; and urology, 2. Consultants, in general, were highly supportive of the linkages (i.e., [1] agreed that they resulted in improvement of patient comfort/satisfaction, [2] reduced risk of adverse outcomes, [3] reduced overall costs, and [4] were important issues for the guidelines to address). Responses were given on a 5-point scale, ranging from 1, strongly disagree, to 5, strongly agree; support for a linkage was defined as the fraction of consultants responding "4" or "5" to a given linkage. The percentage of consultants reporting support for each linkage is reported in Table 2. Additional re-

TABLE 2 *Proportion of Consultants Indicating Support for Linkages*

LINKAGE	PATIENT COMFORT/ SATISFACTION (%)	REDUCED RISK (%)	REDUCED COSTS (%)	IMPORTANT TOPIC (%)
1 (patient evaluation)	57	92	63	62
2 (pre-procedure preparation)	92	85	63	65
3a (level of consciousness)	70	87	52	71
3b (ventilation monitoring— observation/auscultation)	45	85	43	70
3c (automated apnea monitoring)	32	74	30	72
3d (pulse oximetry)	77	96	56	81
3e (heart rate and blood pressure)	55	83	45	66
4 (contemporaneous recording of monitored parameters)	23	67	38	67
5 (staff availability)	58	65	31	75
6 (training of personnel)	69	94	67	77
7 (availability of emergency equipment)	42	96	54	63
8 (supplemental oxygen)	35	50	19	67
9 (multiple agents)	48	13	7	71
10 (titration)	87	81	55	70
11 (IV access)	42	85	33	67
12 (reversal agents)	35	85	29	71
13 (post-procedure monitoring)	67	92	52	81
14a (special regimens)	71	88	37	67
14b (anesthesia consultation)	70	74	34	68

sponses from consultants are listed as follows: (1) percentage of consultants supporting continuous electrocardiographic monitoring of different classes of patients was for all patients, 23%; patients with hypertension, 51%; patients with cardiovascular disease, 91%; and patients with cardiac dysrhythmias, 94%; (2) percentage of consultants supporting the immediate availability of a defibrillator for different classes of patients was for all patients, 64%; patients with hypertension, 68%; patients with cardiovascular disease, 83%; and patients with dysrhythmias, 85%; and (3) percentage of consultants supporting determination of vital signs and respiratory variables at the following times was prior to sedation, 91%; immediately after sedation initiated, 79%; at regular intervals during procedure, 83%; at beginning of recovery, 89%; at intervals during recovery, 81%; and before discharge, 87%.

The feasibility of implementing these guidelines into clinical practice was assessed by an opinion survey of those respondents from the consultant panel who were nonanesthesiologists ($n = 37$). Responses for feasibility of implementation of the guidelines were as follows. Seventy-five percent of these consultants indicated that implementation of the guidelines would not result in the need to purchase new equipment, supplies, or pharmaceuticals. Among the 25% who stated that purchases would be required, the median anticipated cost was $3,750 (mean = $6,167; range = $1,500 to $20,000). Anticipated new costs included hiring and training (e.g., ACLS) of personnel, the presence of a nurse during procedures, establishing IV access as a routine procedure, exhaled CO_2 monitoring equipment, defibrillator, more attention to pre-procedure needs (e.g., NPO status), and additional personnel time during recovery.

The non-anesthesiologist consultants were asked to indicate which, if any, of the evidence linkages would change their clinical practices if the guidelines were instituted. Percentages of consultants expecting no change associated with each linkage were as follows: pre-procedure history, 81%; preparation of the patient, 76%; direct monitoring of patient dedicated staff, 89%; respiration, 89%; automated ventilatory monitoring, 38%; pulse oximetry, 95%; cardiovascular monitoring, 95%; education and training, 95%; emergency equipment, 95%; supplemental oxygen, 95%; multiple classes of agents, 95%; titration, 92%; IV access, 89%; reversal agents, 92%; post-procedure monitoring, 89%; and pre-procedure consultation with an anesthesiologist, 84%.

Sixty-six percent of the respondents indicated that the guidelines would have no effect on the amount of time spent on a typical case. None reported that the guidelines would reduce the amount of time spent per case. For all respondents, the mean increase in the amount of time spent on a typical case was 4.8 minutes. Of the 32% of respondents who reported an anticipated increase in time spent on a typical case, the mean was 14.0 minutes (range = 5.0 to 30.0 minutes).

Readers with special interest in the statistical analyses used in establishing these guidelines can receive further information by writing to: Jeffrey B. Gross, MD, Department of Anesthesiology (M/C 2015), University of Connecticut School of Medicine, Farmington, CT 06030-2015.

APPENDIX 2: DEFINITION OF TERMS

In these guidelines, the following terms are used to express the strength of the evidence relating various interventions and the associated outcomes:

FOR LITERATURE REVIEW

Insufficient data:	There is insufficient published data to provide an indication of the relationship between intervention and outcome.
Suggests:	There is qualitative evidence in the form of case reports or descriptive studies but there is insufficient quantitative evidence to establish a statistical relationship between intervention and outcome.
Supports:	Quantitative data indicate a significant relationship between intervention and outcome ($p < 0.01$), and qualitative data are supportive.

FOR CONSULTANT OPINION

The consultants' questionnaire was based on a 5-point scale ranging from "1" (strongly disagree) to "5" (strongly agree), with a score of "3" being neutral.

Suggests:	The number of individuals responding "4" or "5" exceeds the number responding "1" or "2".
Supports:	50% or more of the responses were "4" or "5."
Strongly supports:	50% or more of the responses were "5."

APPENDIX 3: SUMMARY OF GUIDELINES*

1. Pre-procedure evaluation
   - Relevant history
   - Focused physical exam (to include heart, lungs, airway)
   - Laboratory testing when indicated
2. Patient counseling: risks, benefits, limitations, and alternatives
3. Pre-procedure fasting
   - Elective procedures—sufficient time for gastric emptying
   - Urgent or emergent situations—benefits of sedation/analgesia must be weighed against the potential risk of regurgitation and aspiration of gastric contents.
4. Monitoring (data to be recorded at appropriate intervals before, during, and after procedure)
   - Pulse oximetry
   - Response to verbal commands when practical

---

*This is a summary of the guidelines. The body of the document should be consulted for complete details.

- Pulmonary ventilation (observation, auscultation, other means)
- Blood pressure and heart rate at appropriate intervals
- Electrocardiograph for patients with significant cardiovascular disease

5. Personnel: designated individual, other than the practitioner performing the procedure, present to monitor the patient throughout the procedure

6. Training
   - Pharmacology of sedative and analgesic agents
   - Pharmacology of available antagonists
   - Basic life support skills—present
   - Advanced life support skills—immediately available

7. Emergency equipment
   - Suction, appropriately sized airway equipment, means of positive-pressure ventilation intravenous equipment, pharmacologic antagonists, and basic resuscitative medications

8. Supplemental oxygen
   - Oxygen delivery equipment available
   - Oxygen administered if hypoxemia occurs

9. Choice of agents
   - Sedatives to decrease anxiety, promote somnolence
   - Analgesics to relieve pain

10. Dose titration
    - Medications given incrementally with sufficient time between doses to assess effects
    - Appropriate dose reduction if both sedatives and analgesics used

11. Intravenous access
    - Sedatives administered intravenously—maintain IV access
    - Sedatives administered by other routes—case-by-case decision

12. Recovery
    - Observation until patients no longer at risk for cardiorespiratory depression
    - Appropriate discharge criteria

13. Special situations
    - Severe underlying medical problems—consult with appropriate specialist
    - Risk of severe cardiovascular or respiratory compromise or need for deep sedation/general anesthesia to obtain adequate operating conditions—consult anesthesiologist

Association of Operating Room Nurses Recommended Practices for Managing the Patient Receiving Conscious Sedation/Analgesia*

The following recommended practices were developed by the Association of Operating Room Nurses (AORN) Recommended Practices Committee and have been approved by the AORN Board of Directors. They were published as proposed recommended practices through the AORN fax-on-demand for comments by members and others. They were effective January 1, 1997.

These recommended practices are intended as achievable recommended practices representing what is believed to be an optimal level of practice. Policies and procedures will reflect variations in practice settings and/or clinical situations that determine the degree to which the recommended practices can be implemented.

AORN recognizes the numerous types of settings in which perioperative nurses practice. These recommended practices are intended as guidelines adaptable to various practice settings. These practice settings include traditional ORs, ambulatory surgery units, physicians' offices, cardiac catheterization laboratories, endoscopy suites, radiology departments, and all other areas where surgery may be performed.

PURPOSE

Sedation and analgesia describes a state which allows patients to tolerate unpleasant procedures while maintaining adequate cardiorespiratory function and the ability to respond purposefully to verbal command and/or tactile stimulation. Patients whose only response is reflex withdrawal from a painful stimulus are sedated to a greater degree than encompassed by sedation/analgesia. (American Society of Anesthesiologists, 1995.)

These recommended practices provide guidelines for RNs managing patients receiving conscious sedation/analgesia. Patient selection for conscious sedation/analgesia should be based on established criteria developed through interdisciplinary collaboration of health care professionals. The type of monitoring used with patients who receive conscious sedation/analgesia, the medications selected, and the interventions taken must be within the defined scope of perioperative nursing practice.

Certain patients are not candidates for conscious sedation/analgesia with monitoring by RNs. These patients may require more extensive monitoring and sedation, as provided by anesthesia care providers, and should be identified in consultation with anesthesiologists, surgeons, and other physicians. It is not the intent of these recommended practices to address situations that require the services of anesthesia care providers.

The patient care and monitoring guidelines in these recommended practices may be exceeded at any time. Their intent is to encourage quality patient care; however, implementation of these recommended practices cannot guarantee specific patient outcomes. These recommended practices are subject to revision as warranted by advances in nursing practice and technology.

RECOMMENDED PRACTICE I

RNs should understand the goals and objectives of conscious sedation/analgesia.

INTERPRETIVE STATEMENT 1

The primary goal of conscious sedation/analgesia is to reduce the patient's anxiety and discomfort so as to facilitate cooperation between the patient and the caregivers. Conscious sedation/analgesia can be used as an adjunct to local anesthesia during the procedure.

RATIONALE

Adequate preoperative preparation and verbal reassurances from RNs facilitate the desired effects of conscious sedation/analgesia and may allow for a decrease of the dosages of opioids, benzodiazepines, and sedatives used (Watson & James, 1990).

INTERPRETIVE STATEMENT 2

Objectives for the patient receiving conscious sedation/analgesia include:
- Alteration of mood
- Maintenance of consciousness
- Enhanced cooperation
- Elevation of the pain threshold
- Minimal variation of vital signs
- Some degree of amnesia
- A rapid, safe return to activities of daily living

RATIONALE

Conscious sedation/analgesia produces a condition in which the patient exhibits a depressed level of consciousness but retains the ability to independently respond appropriately to verbal commands or physical stimulation. Misunderstanding the objectives of conscious sedation/analgesia may jeopardize the quality of patient care (Position statement, 1992; Watson & James, 1990).

RECOMMENDED PRACTICE II

The RN monitoring the patient who receives conscious sedation/analgesia should have no other responsibilities that would require the nurse to leave the patient unattended or compromise continuous patient monitoring during the procedure.

INTERPRETIVE STATEMENT 1

The RN should provide continuous monitoring of the patient who receives conscious sedation/analgesia. The RN must be able to immediately recognize and respond to adverse physiologic and psychologic changes during the procedure.

RATIONALE

It is unrealistic to assume that one RN can perform circulating duties and also provide continuous monitoring, physical care, and emotional support for the patient who receives conscious sedation/analgesia (Position statement, 1992; Watson & James, 1990).

RECOMMENDED PRACTICE III

The RN monitoring the patient's care should be clinically competent in the function and in the use of resuscitation medications and monitoring equipment and be able to interpret the data obtained from the patient.

INTERPRETIVE STATEMENT 1

The RN who is monitoring the patient should understand how to operate monitoring equipment used during conscious sedation/analgesia.

RATIONALE

Knowledge of the function and proper use of monitoring equipment is essential for providing safe patient care (Watson & James, 1990).

INTERPRETIVE STATEMENT 2

The nurse who is monitoring the patient should demonstrate knowledge of:
- Anatomy and physiology
- Pharmacology of medications used for conscious sedation/analgesia
- Cardiac arrhythmia interpretation
- Possible complications related to the use of conscious sedation/analgesia
- Respiratory functions (i.e., oxygen delivery, transport, uptake)

RATIONALE

Medications used for conscious sedation/analgesia may cause rapid, adverse physiologic responses in the patient. Early detection of such responses allows for rapid intervention and treatment (Watson & James, 1990).

INTERPRETIVE STATEMENT 3

The RN who is monitoring the patient should be competent in the use of oxygen delivery devices and airway management.

RATIONALE

Rapid intervention is necessary in the event of complications from the undesired effects of conscious sedation/analgesia (Watson & James, 1990).

DISCUSSION

The airway management skill level of the RN who is monitoring the patient receiving conscious sedation/analgesia should be defined by the health care facility's policies and procedures. Basic cardiac life support, which includes maintenance of the patient's airway by use of the head-tilt or chin-lift maneuver, is considered a basic competency for all RNs. The use of oxygen delivery devices (e.g., respirator bag, face mask device) may be included as part of the orientation and continuing education process for RNs who monitor patients receiving conscious sedation/analgesia. Advanced cardiac life support (ACLS) certification may be required in some health care facilities. Health care professionals with ACLS skills (e.g., ACLS team members, anesthesia care providers) should be readily available to every location in which conscious sedation/analgesia is being administered.

INTERPRETIVE STATEMENT 4

Health care facilities should provide competency-based educational programs for all RNs who manage patients undergoing conscious sedation/analgesia. These programs should offer a variety of learning opportunities based on learners' needs.

RATIONALE

The facility should have an educational/competency validation mechanism in place that includes a process for evaluating and documenting RNs' demonstration of knowledge, skills, and abilities related to the management of patients receiving conscious sedation/analgesia. Evaluation and documentation of competence should occur on a periodic basis according to the health care facility's policies and procedures (Position statement, 1992).

RECOMMENDED PRACTICE IV

Each patient who will receive conscious sedation/analgesia should be assessed physiologically and psychologically before the procedure. The assessment should be documented in the patient's record.

INTERPRETIVE STATEMENT 1

A preprocedure patient assessment should include a review of:
- Physical examination findings
- Current medications
- Drug allergies/sensitivities
- Current medical problems (e.g., hypertension, diabetes, cardiopulmonary disease, liver disease, renal disease)
- Tobacco smoking and substance abuse history
- Chief complaint
- Baseline vital signs, including height, weight, and age
- Level of consciousness
- Emotional state
- Communication ability
- Perceptions regarding procedure and conscious sedation/analgesia

RATIONALE

A preprocedure assessment provides health care professionals baseline data and identifies the patient's risk factors (Kidwell, 1991; Watson & James, 1990).

RECOMMENDED PRACTICE V

Each patient who receives conscious sedation/analgesia should be monitored for adverse reactions to medications and for physiologic and psychologic changes.

INTERPRETIVE STATEMENT 1

The RN who administers medications for conscious sedation/analgesia should be responsible for understanding the medications:
- Indications and dosages
- Contraindications
- Adverse reactions and emergency management techniques
- Interactions with other medications
- Onset and duration of action
- Desired effects

RATIONALE

Patient anxiety and medications used for conscious sedation/analgesia may cause rapid, adverse physiologic and psychologic changes in the patient (Watson & James, 1990).

INTERPRETIVE STATEMENT 2

The RN who monitors the patient receiving conscious sedation/analgesia should be knowledgeable of the desirable and undesirable medication effects of conscious sedation/analgesia.

RATIONALE

Observation of the patient for desired therapeutic medication effects, prevention of avoidable medication reactions, early detection and management of unexplained adverse reaction, and accurate documentation of the patient's response are integral components of the monitoring process (Kidwell, 1991; Watson & James, 1990).

DISCUSSION

Desirable effects of conscious sedation/analgesia include:
- Intact protective reflexes
- Relaxation
- Comfort
- Cooperation
- Diminished verbal communication
- Patent airway with adequate ventilatory exchange
- Easy arousal from sleep

Potential complications of conscious sedation/analgesia include:
- Aspiration
- Severely slurred speech
- Unarousable sleep
- Hypotension
- Agitation
- Combativeness
- Hypoventilation
- Respiratory depression
- Airway obstruction
- Apnea

INTERPRETIVE STATEMENT 3

Before conscious sedation is administered, an oxygen delivery device should be in place or immediately available, an intravenous access line should be established, and appropriate monitoring devices should be in place.

RATIONALE

Sedatives and benzodiazepines used for conscious sedation/analgesia may cause somnolence, confusion, coma, diminished reflexes, and depressed respiratory and cardiovascular functions. Opioids used for conscious sedation/analgesia may cause respiratory depression, hypotension, nausea, and vomiting. Overdosage and adverse reactions may occur any time during the procedure and may be reversible (Watson & James, 1990).

DISCUSSION

The following equipment should be present and ready for use in the room in which conscious sedation/analgesia is administered:

- Oxygen
- Suction apparatus
- Oxygen delivery devices
- Noninvasive blood pressure device
- Electrocardiograph
- Pulse oximeter

Monitoring parameters should include:

- Respiratory rate
- Oxygen saturation
- Blood pressure
- Cardiac rate and rhythm
- Level of consciousness
- Skin condition

Undesirable changes in patient condition should be reported immediately to the physician.

INTERPRETIVE STATEMENT 4

Each patient who receives conscious sedation/analgesia intravenously should have continuous intravenous access. If medications are not administered intravenously, the need for intravenous access should be determined on a case-by-case basis. In all instances, an individual with the skills to establish intravenous access should be immediately available.

RATIONALE

Continuous intravenous access provides a means for administering medications used for conscious sedation/analgesia and for implementing emergency medications and fluids to counteract adverse medication effects (Kidwell, 1991).

DISCUSSION

Continuous intravenous access may be obtained using an intravenous access device or by infusing intravenous fluids through an access port. The type of continuous intravenous access chosen will vary depending on health care facilities' policies and procedures and physicians' preferences.

INTERPRETIVE STATEMENT 5

An emergency cart with appropriate resuscitative medications, including narcotic and sedative reversal medications, and equipment (e.g., defibrillator) should be immediately available to every location in which conscious sedation/analgesia is being administered.

RATIONALE

Medication overdoses or adverse reactions may cause respiratory depression, hypotension, or impaired cardiovascular function requiring immediate intervention or cardiopulmonary resuscitation (CPR) (Watson & James, 1990). Equipment for CPR or emergency medication reversals should be available for immediate use because diminished reflexes, depressed respiratory function, and impaired cardiovascular function may occur within seconds or minutes after the administration of medications used for conscious sedation/analgesia (Bailey et al., 1990; Position statement, 1992).

RECOMMENDED PRACTICE VI

Documentation of patient care during conscious sedation should be consistent with the AORN "Recommended Practices for Documentation of Perioperative Nursing Care" wherever conscious sedation/analgesia is administered.

INTERPRETIVE STATEMENT 1

Nursing diagnoses applicable to patients receiving conscious sedation/analgesia may include the potential for:
- Anxiety related to the unfamiliar environment and procedure
- Ineffective breathing patterns or impaired gas exchange related to altered level of consciousness or airway obstruction
- Knowledge deficit related to poor recall resulting from medication effects
- Cardiac output changes related to medication effects on the myocardium
- Injury related to altered level of consciousness

RATIONALE

Use of nursing diagnoses for planning the care of patients who receive conscious sedation/analgesia provides for patient care that focuses on patients' responses to the procedure or nursing interventions. Nursing interventions are directed toward positive patient outcomes (Kleinbeck, 1990).

INTERPRETIVE STATEMENT 2

Documentation should include:
- Preprocedure assessment
- Dosage, route, time, and effects of all medications and fluids used
- Type and amount of fluids administered, including blood and blood products, monitoring devices, and equipment used
- Physiologic data from continuous monitoring at 5- to 15-minute intervals and upon significant events

- Level of consciousness
- Nursing interventions taken and the patient's responses
- Untoward significant patient reactions and their resolution

RATIONALE

Documentation of nursing interventions promotes continuity of patient care and improves communication among health care team members. Documentation also provides a mechanism for comparing actual versus expected patient outcomes (AORN, 1996).

RECOMMENDED PRACTICE VII

Patients who receive conscious sedation/analgesia should be monitored postprocedure, receive verbal and written discharge instructions, and meet specified criteria before discharge.

DISCUSSION

Postprocedure patient care, monitoring, and discharge criteria should be consistent for all patients. Patients and their family members or caregivers should receive verbal and written discharge instructions and verbalize an understanding of the instructions to the nurse. Preprocedure and postprocedure instructions, as well as verbalization of understanding, is encouraged because medications used for conscious sedation/analgesia may cause significant patient amnesia that directly affects recall ability (Watson & James, 1990).

Discharge guidelines provide specific criteria for assessing and evaluating the patient's readiness for discharge and home care. Discharge criteria should reflect indications that the patient has returned to a safe physiologic level. These indicators should include:

- Adequate respiratory function
- Stability of vital signs, including temperature
- Preprocedure level of consciousness
- Intact protective reflexes
- Return of motor/sensory control
- Absence of protracted nausea
- Skin color and condition
- Satisfactory surgical site and dressing condition, when present
- Absence of significant pain (American Society of Post-Anesthesia Nurses, 1995).

The presence of a responsible adult escort is necessary for discharge. Discharge criteria should be developed by representatives from the medical staff, anesthesia, nursing, and other departments as appropriate.

RECOMMENDED PRACTICE VIII

Policies and procedures for managing patients who receive conscious sedation/analgesia should be written, reviewed periodically, and readily available within the practice setting.

DISCUSSION

Policies and procedures for managing patients receiving conscious sedation/analgesia should include:
- Patient selection criteria
- Extent of and responsibility for monitoring
- Method of recording patient data
- Data to be documented
- Frequency of the patient's physiologic data documentation
- Medications that may be administered by the RN
- Discharge criteria

Policies and procedures are operational guidelines that are used to minimize patient risk factors, standardize practice, assist staff members, and establish guidelines for continuous quality improvement activities by establishing authority, responsibility, and accountability.

GLOSSARY

Benzodiazepines: A pharmacologic family of central nervous system depressants possessing anxiolytic, hypnotic, and skeletal muscle–relaxant properties. These medications are used to allay anxiety and fear and produce varying amnesic effects during conscious sedation/analgesia. Diazepam and midazolam are two benzodiazepines commonly used for conscious sedation/analgesia.

Conscious sedation/analgesia: A minimally depressed level of consciousness that allows a surgical patient to retain the ability to independently and continuously maintain a patent airway and respond appropriately to verbal commands and physical stimulation.

Managing the patient: The use of nursing process to deliver and direct comprehensive nursing care during a procedure in a practice setting.

Monitoring: Clinical observation that is individualized to patient needs based on data obtained from preprocedure patient assessments. The objective of monitoring patients who receive conscious sedation is to improve patient outcomes. Monitoring includes the use of mechanical devices and direct observation.

Opioid: Natural or synthetic pharmacologic agents that produce varying degrees of analgesia and sedation and relieve pain. Fentanyl and meperidine hydrochloride are two opioid analgesic medications that may be used for conscious sedation/analgesia.

Sedatives: Pharmacologic agents that reduce anxiety and may induce some degree of short-term amnesia.

REFERENCES

American Association of Operating Room Nurses (1996). Recommended practices for documentation of perioperative nursing care. In *AORN standards and recommended practices.* Denver: Author.

American Society of Anesthesiologists (1995). *Guidelines for sedation and analgesia by non-anesthesiologists.* Park Ridge, IL: Author.

American Society of Post-Anesthesia Nurses (1995). *Standards of perianesthesia nursing practice: 1996.* Thorofare, NJ: Author.

Bailey, P.L., et al. (1990). Frequent hypoxemia and apnea after sedation with midazolam and fentanyl. *Anesthesiology 73,* 826-830.

Kidwell, J.A. (1991). Nursing care for the patient receiving conscious sedation during gastrointestinal endoscopic procedures. *Gastroenterology Nursing 13,* 136-137.

Kleinbeck, S.V.M. (1990). Introduction to the nursing process. In J.C. Rothrock (Ed.), *Perioperative nursing care planning.* St Louis: Mosby.

Position statement on the role of the RN in the management of patients receiving IV conscious sedation for short-term therapeutic, diagnostic, or surgical procedures (1992). *AORN Journal 55,* 207.

Watson, D.S., James, D.S. (1990). Intravenous conscious sedation: Implications of monitoring patients receiving local anesthesia. *AORN Journal 51,* 1513-1522.

SUGGESTED READING

American Association of Nurse Anesthetists (1983). *American Association of Nurse Anesthetists guidelines for practice of the certified registered nurse anesthetist.* Park Ridge IL: Author.

Index

Oxygen—cont'd
  myocardial ischemia and, 86
  supplemental, 230
Oxygen saturation, 31-33
  respiratory complications and, 82
Oxygenation, monitoring of, 227
Oxyhemoglobin dissociation curve, 32

P

Pain
  anxiety and, 77
  chest, 86
  in child, 142
  mechanical ventilation and, 159-160, 181
Pain threshold, 16
Palate, soft, 22
Palpation, chest, 34
Paradoxical reaction to drug, 77
Partial pressure of arterial oxygen, 31, 32
  aspiration treatment and, 81
Partial pressure of carbon dioxide, 31-32
Patient discharge, 97-106
Patient management, competence in, 130-131
Pediatric sedation, 141-157
  assessment in
    intraprocedure, 146-147
    postprocedure, 147
    preprocedure, 144-146
  drug administration for, 147-152, 153
  guidelines for, 142-144
  standard of care for, 154-157
Percussion, 34
Personnel training, 229
Pharmacology, 43-68; *see also* Drug
Phenothiazines, drug interactions with, 26
Phenylephrine, 85
Phone call, postprocedure, 103, 106
Physical evaluation, preprocedural, 21-25
Physical status classification, 20
Piggybacked intravenous administration, 44
Planning, discharge, 97-106; *see also* Discharge
    of patient
Pneumothorax, 180
Policy and guideline development, 107-124; *see
    also* Standards
Popliteal pulse, 29
Position statement, 10, 213-215
Posterior tibial pulse, 29
Postprocedure assessment, 38-40, 98-100
Postprocedure care, 232-233
Postprocedure phone call, 103, 106
Practice guidelines, 10-11, 72-73
Practice standards, 5, 8-13, 245-254
Premature beat, ventricular, 87
Preprocedure assessment, 19-27; *see also* As-
    sessment, preprocedure
Professional organization
  development of care standards and, 13
  practice standards and, 5, 8-13
Propofol
  half-life of, 172
  mechanical ventilation and, 171, 176-177
  pharmacology of, 65-67
Psychologic factors
  assessment of, 21
  for child, 142
  mechanical ventilation and, 159

Psychosis
  drugs for, 166-180
    combination therapy with, 179
    neuroleptic, 177-179
    opioid, 168-177
    tolerance to, 179-180
  pathophysiology of, 160-166
Pulmonary complications, 78-79
Pulse
  arrhythmia and, 88
  intraprocedural monitoring of, 28-33
Pulse oximetry, 82-83
Pulseless electrical activity, 88
Push, intravenous, 43

R

Ramsay sedation scale, 37-38, 182-183, 184
Recommended practices, 12
Record of monitored parameters, 228
Recovery care, 232-233
Rectal sedation in child, 148, 152
Reflex, 16
Renal disease, 24
Report, nurse's, 97-98
Resedation, 54, 90
Respiration monitoring, 33-35
Respiratory complications, 78-79
Respiratory disorder, history of, 23
Respiratory distress
  in adult, 180-181
  in child, 146
Respiratory insufficiency, 82-83
Reversal agent
  benzodiazepine, 53-55, 89-91
  mechanical ventilation and, 189
  opioid, 64-65, 91-93
  recommendations for, 231-232
Revex, 92
Rhythm, pulse, 30
Risk factors, for aspiration, in child, 145-146
Rival; *see* Diazepam
Romazicon; *see* Flumazenil
Roxanol; *see* Morphine

S

Saturation, oxygen, 31-33
  respiratory complications and, 82
Scale
  conscious sedation, 37-38, 39, 182-185
  postanesthesia, 99, 100
Scope of nursing practice, 5-13
Sedation scale, 37-38, 39, 182-185
Seizure disorder, history of, 23
Shelly sedation scale, 184, 185
Skill-based competence, 133
Soft palate, airway evaluation and, 22
Stadol, 58-59
Standards
  of care, 107-124
    for basic anesthetic monitoring, 209-212
    benchmarks for, 113, 119
    for child, 154-157
    communication and, 119
    Duke University policy and, 120-124
    evaluation form for, 114
    evaluation of national standards and, 113
    Harris County Hospital policy and, 109-112,
      115-117

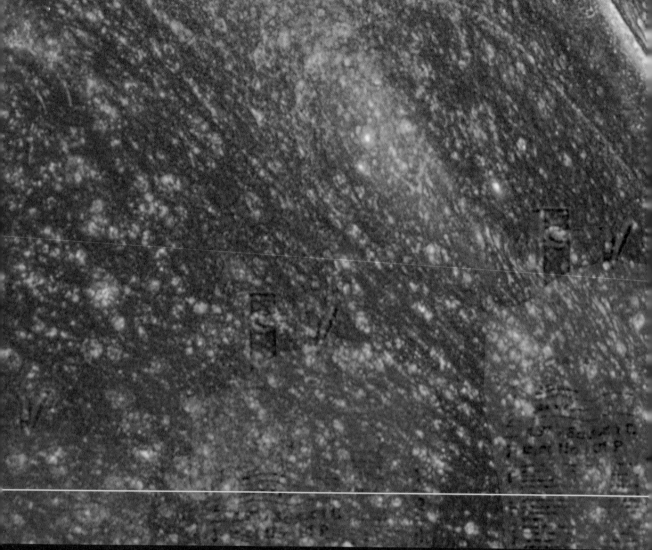

M Mosby

ISBN 0-8151-9265-7

9 780815 192657

90000

27471